DSM-III
TRAINING GUIDE

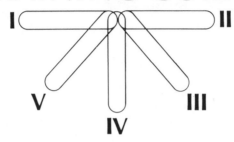

DSM-III
TRAINING GUIDE

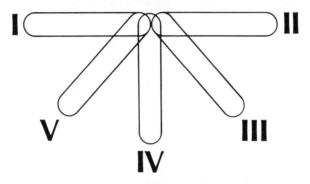

For Use with the
American Psychiatric Association's
Diagnostic and Statistical Manual
of Mental Disorders (Third Edition)

Editors

Linda J. Webb, Dr. P. H.,
Carlo C. DiClemente, Ph.D.,
Edwin E. Johnstone, M.D.,
Joyce L. Sanders, R. N., M.S.H.P., and
Robin A. Perley, M.P.H.

Office of Continuing Education
Texas Department of Mental Health and Mental Retardation
Texas Research Institute of Mental Sciences

Brunner/Mazel, *Publishers* • New York

Library of Congress Cataloging in Publication Data

Main entry under title:

DSM-III training guide for use with the American Psychiatric Association's Diagnostic
   and statistical manual of mental disorders (third edition).

   1. Psychology, Pathological—Classification.   2. Psychology, Pathological—Diagnosis.
I. Webb, Linda J.   II. Texas Research Institute of Mental Sciences.   Office of Continuing
Education.   III. Diagnostic and statistical manual of mental disorders. 3rd ed.
[DNLM: 1.   Mental Disorders—Classification.   2.   Psychiatry—Nomenclature.
WM   15   A5123d 1980 Suppl.]
RC455.2.C4D75   1981   616.89′075   81-10174
                                            AACR2

Clothbound edition ISBN 0-87630-279-7
Paperbound edition ISBN 0-87630-293-2

Foreword

In teaching DSM-III at numerous workshops, we have often been asked by those responsible for teaching the new classification at their own institutions whether an outline of DSM-III was available to assist in the preparation of lectures. Recognizing the value of such a teaching guide, we started to prepare one ourselves. We soon realized that in order to do it well, a great deal of time and effort was necessary, and under the pressure of other activities, we abandoned the project (bogged down, as we recall, in the mire of Major Depression).

Fortunately, little known to us, the Office of Continuing Education, Texas Department of Mental Health and Mental Retardation, Texas Research Institute of Mental Sciences (TRIMS) had the same idea, as well as the endurance and technical know-how to complete the project. Not only have they outlined DSM-III with great care, but they have also prepared a comprehensive set of slides that will be of great value to anyone wishing to teach one or more sections of DSM-III. Also included in their package are several videotaped vignettes for practice in applying DSM-III to clinical material.

In preparing these materials, TRIMS has performed a significant service for the mental health professions.

ROBERT L. SPITZER, M.D.
ANDREW E. SKODOL, M.D.
JANET B. W. WILLIAMS, M.S.W.
MIRIAM GIBBON, M.S.W.

Contents

SECTION III   Review of Major Classifications

SECTION IV   Application

Preface

In the Spring of 1980 the Office of Continuing Education, Texas Department of Mental Health and Mental Retardation, Texas Research Institute of Mental Sciences, initiated a training program to train professionals in the Texas Department of Mental Health and Mental Retardation in the concepts and use of the American Psychiatric Association's Diagnostic and Statistical Manual of Mental Disorders, Third Edition (DSM-III). Multidisciplinary training teams, consisting of a psychiatrist, psychologist, social worker, nurse, staff development specialist, and medical records administrator, from each of the Department's state hospitals, schools, and community centers, were trained at regional workshops.

The workshops were designed to train the teams of trainers in the basic concepts and use of DSM-III and to prepare them to train the professionals in their own facilities. To assist the training teams, a training package consisting of a Training Guide, a set of accompanying slides, and a videotape cassette with five case vignettes, was developed by a multidisciplinary faculty at the Texas Research Institute of Mental Sciences. These educational materials enabled the teams to return to their respective institutions and to train, with some uniformity, the mental health and mental retardation professionals throughout the Department.

After considerable success with the training program and numerous requests from other organizations and individuals, the Office of Continuing Education decided to make the training materials available to the general public. Dr. Robert Spitzer and his colleagues, Dr. Andrew Skodol, Janet Williams, and Miriam Gibbon, very generously agreed to review and critique the Training Guide, slides, and videotape. Based on their comments and recommendations, as well as our experience with the training program, numerous revisions were made in the original materials.

As a result, this new and, we believe, considerably improved edition of the Training Guide is now available to individuals as a self-instruction guide, and to institutions for use in conjunction with the slides and videotape to train the professionals in their organizations.

The Training Guide, in conjunction with the DSM-III manual, can be used by individuals for in-depth study and review of diagnostic classifications and to prepare them to accurately apply the new DSM-III classification system to the diagnosis of their clients/patients.

The DSM-III Training Program for Health Professionals consists of the Training Guide, an accompanying set of slides, and a videotape with five case vignettes. These training materials are designed for educators to teach students and train professionals from various disciplines. The Training Program is ideally suited for universities, medical schools, state departments of mental health and other organizations of sufficient size to require in-house training in the use of DSM-III. These materials have proven to be effective for training multidisciplinary groups as well as for discipline specific subgroups, i.e. psychiatrists, psychologists, social workers, nurses, and other related mental health and mental retardation professionals (Webb et al., 1981).

ACKNOWLEDGMENTS

The DSM-III Training Program for Health Professionals was developed with the assistance of many people. The curriculum authors, listed under contributors, not only prepared their respective chapters but were involved in the conceptualization of the original Training Guide and the design of the DSM-III Training Program for Health Professionals in the Texas Department of Mental Health and Mental Retardation. To list them as contributors does not begin to acknowledge the extraordinarily generous commitment of their time and effort.

Likewise, the editors' diligent revisions of the original Training Guide and slides have contributed substantially to the improved clarity and, it is hoped, utility of the Training Program. Without Drs. Carlos DiClemente's and Ed Johnstone's work on revising the content, this Training Guide would not have been possible. Likewise, Joyce Sanders' careful attention to editorial detail and slide revisions, and Robin Perley's persistent efforts at organizing and editing the Guide were invaluable.

Dr. Robert L. Spitzer and his colleagues, Dr. Andrew E. Skodol, Janet B. W. Williams, and Miriam Gibbon very generously donated their time to reviewing the original Guide and recommending revisions.

Mildred Dobson, Sherol Zuniga, and Ira Mae Sam's tireless efforts at typing and xeroxing revision after revision, plus their good humor and support, were essential to the completion of the project.

Mike McGuyer and his staff, Peter Baer, Marcus Meyers and Kathleen Mulkey, in the Audiovisual Section, Texas Research Institute of Mental Sciences, were responsible for the development of the videotape and slides that accompanied the original Guide. Mike, along with Joyce L. Sanders, was also responsible for the revision of the slides.

Dr. Dave Culclasure, Lynn Wade, Robert Eardley, and their staff at San Antonio State Hospital very generously contracted to revise the original slides and produced the set that accompanies this Training Guide.

Recognition should be given to Dr. John Kavanagh, Commissioner, Texas Department of Mental Health and Mental Retardation; Dr. Joseph Schoolar, Director, Texas Research Institute of Mental Sciences; and Dr. James Claghorn, Assistant Director, Texas Research Institute of Mental Sciences, for their support in the development of the original training package and encouragement to nationally publish the Training Program.

Appreciation is also expressed to the professionals in the Texas Department of Mental Health and Mental Retardation who participated in the original training program. Their evaluation and critique of the program contributed substantially in helping us revise and improve the DSM-III Training Program for Health Professionals.

And finally, there have been numerous others at the Texas Research Institute of Mental Sciences who have contributed to the development of the Training Program. While it is not possible to list them all, a special word of thanks is given to them for their support.

LINDA J. WEBB, DR.P.H.
Director, Office of Continuing Education
Texas Department of Mental Health and
Mental Retardation
Texas Research Institute of Mental Sciences

Contributors

Linda Bond, B.S., R.R.A., Chief, Quality Assurance, St. Joseph's Hospital, Houston, Texas (Chapter 23)

James L. Claghorn, M.D., Assistant Director and Chief, Training Division, Texas Research Institute of Mental Sciences, Houston, Texas (Chapters 1, 2)

Carlo C. DiClemente, Ph.D., Clinical Psychologist, Adult Outpatient Services, Texas Research Institute of Mental Sciences, Houston, Texas (Chapters 9, 13, 14, 15, 16, 21, 22, 23, 24)

James Ganc, M.D., Chief, Children's Clinic, Texas Research Institute of Mental Sciences, Houston, Texas (Chapter 9)

Mary Beth Holley, M.S.W., Assistant Chief, Adolescent and Family Clinic, Texas Research Institute of Mental Sciences, Houston, Texas (Chapter 16)

Edwin E. Johnstone, M.D., Director, Psychiatric Residency Training Program, Texas Research Institute of Mental Sciences, Houston, Texas (Chapters 3, 4, 5, 6, 10, 11, 12, 24)

Mohsen Mirabi, M.D., Chief, Adult Outpatient Department, Texas Research Institute of Mental Sciences, Houston, Texas (Chapters 5, 6, 12)

Robin A. Perley, M.P.H., Office of Continuing Education, Texas Department of Mental Health and Mental Retardation, Texas Research Institute of Mental Sciences, Houston, Texas (Chapter 24)

Joyce L. Sanders, R. N., M.S.H.P., Assistant Director, Office of Continuing Education, Texas Department of Mental Health and Mental Retardation, Texas Research Institute of Mental Sciences, Houston, Texas (Chapters 1, 2, 17, 18, 19, 20)

Joseph C. Schoolar, Ph.D., M.D., Director, Texas Research Institute of Mental Sciences, Houston, Texas (Chapters 1, 2)

Kenneth S. Solway, Ph.D., Section Chief, Clinical Psychology and Social Services Training Section, Texas Research Institute of Mental Sciences, Houston, Texas (Chapter 9)

Linda J. Webb, Dr.P.H., Director, Office of Continuing Education, Texas Department of Mental Health and Mental Retardation, Texas Research Institute of Mental Sciences, Houston, Texas (Introduction, Chapters 7, 8)

CONSULTANTS
Robert L. Spitzer, M.D., Biometrics Research Department, New York State Psychiatric Institute, New York, New York

Andrew E. Skodol, M.D., Biometrics Research Department, New York State Psychiatric Institute, New York, New York

Janet B. W. Williams, M.S.W., Biometrics Research Department, New York State Psychiatric Institute, New York, New York

Miriam Gibbon, M.S.W., Biometrics Research Department, New York State Psychiatric Institute, New York, New York

Introduction

The American Psychiatric Association has recommended that effective July 1, 1980, the psychiatric community adopt the long-awaited Diagnostic and Statistical Manual, Third Edition (DSM-III). Because DSM-III is different in many ways from its predecessor, DSM-II, there is a need for continuing education and training of both professionals and students in psychiatry, psychology, social work, nursing and other mental health related professions. The Training Guide provides a detailed outline of the basic concepts of DSM-III and is designed for use by both individuals and institutions.

Individually, the Guide can be used to review the major diagnostic classifications and to prepare for the nosology section of state boards, licensures, and certification examinations. Also, used in conjunction with the DSM-III, the Guide can assist the clinician in accurately applying the new classification system to the diagnosis of patients and clients.

Institutionally, the Training Guide can be used by educators as an instructional guide to teach students and train professionals in the basic concepts and use of DSM-III. A set of accompanying slides and a videotape with five case vignettes are available for institutional purposes. The audiovisuals are designed as a complement to the Guide and provide the educator with supplementary instructional material to train the professionals and students in their organizations. The numbers in the lefthand margin of the Guide refer to the slides. The material included in the slides is also covered in the text of the Guide. Likewise, the five videotape vignettes are described in sufficient detail in Chapter 24 to allow practice in the use of the DSM-III on all five axes.

The Training Guide is divided into four sections with a total of 24 chapters. The first three sections are comprehensive instructional guides and are designed sequentially with each section building on the preceding one. The fourth section addresses the application of the content covered in the first three sections.

Section I reviews the history and development of DSM-III and provides an overview of the multiaxial scheme. The purpose and rationale for DSM-III, the major differences between DSM-II and DSM-III, and the relationship between the mental disorders section of ICD-9-CM and DSM-III are outlined. The rationale for each axis is provided, along with practice examples in its use.

Section II reviews information on the key concepts involved in using DSM-III, such as the glossary, format, decision trees and diagnostic criteria. An introductory overview of the major classifications on Axes I and II is provided, along with a discussion of the use of Axes I and II together. Significant differences between DSM-II and III in the major classifications are outlined. The purpose and the rationale for the use of Axis III is identified and the relationship between Axis III and ICD-9 (Physical Disorders Section) is defined. The purpose and use of Axes IV and V are also described and case vignettes are provided for practice in the use of both Axes IV and V.

Section III provides an in-depth review of specific disorders within the major classifications on Axes I and II and key differences in the DSM-II and DSM-III approaches to the classification. Written case vignettes are included following the review of each major classification with the answers provided in the Appendix of the Guide. Chapters 9 through 22 review each major classification on Axes I and II. Chapter 10 combines Substance Use Disorders and Organic Mental Disorders, since in both classifications factors other than strictly "functional" processes are involved, and it is very often the case that an Organic Mental Disorder is encountered as a consequence of a Substance Use Disorder. Likewise, Chapter 11 combines Schizophrenic Disorders, Paranoid Disorders, and Psychotic Disorders Not Elsewhere Classified because many of these conditions are quite similar on cross-section and can only be distinguished by longitudinal differences.

Section IV is concerned with the application of the information presented in the preceding sections. Chapter 23 includes information on coding procedures, use of fifth digit, and V Codes and E Codes. In Chapter 24 five case vignettes are included to allow practice on all five axes. A discussion follows each of the cases and the answers are included in the Appendix.

While the Guide is organized in a sequential manner, the curriculum may be used in a variety of ways, depending on the learning needs of the particular organization or individual. For example, Section III includes detailed instructional material on each of the major classifications of DSM-III and the specific disorders within the classifications. Some individuals or institutions may want to devote considerable time to reviewing the information on three or four of the major classifications and only briefly review the remaining diagnostic classifications. Others may prefer to study the detailed outline provided on each of the classifications. The users will need to carefully review the content of the Guide and then, depending on their learning needs or the needs of their audience, adapt the materials to meet their educational objectives.

In summary, it is important to emphasize that the Training Guide should be used in conjunction with the DSM-III manual. To be able to accurately apply the multiaxial diagnosis to actual clients/patients, the individual will need not only a good instructional program, but also considerable practice with DSM-III. Likewise, educators who plan to use the Training Program should be familiar with the Training Guide, slides, videotape and, equally important, DSM-III.

DSM-III
TRAINING GUIDE

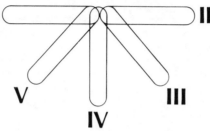

Section I

General Overview

Chapter 1

History and Development

BACKGROUND AND HISTORY

1 Psychiatric nosology dates as far back as 2600 B.C. when the syndromes of melancholia and hysteria appear in the Sumerian and Egyptian literature. From that time until now, such men as Hippocrates, Sydenham, Pinel and Kraepelin have attempted to describe and classify mental disorders.

The first official system for tabulating mental disorders in this country was used for the decennial census in 1840. It contained only one category for all mental disorders and lumped together the idiotic and the insane. In the census of 1880, 40 years later, mental disorders were subdivided into seven categories: mania, melancholia, monomania, paresis, dementia, dispsomania and epilepsy.

2 Today, 100 years later, DSM-III includes 18 major classifications and more than 200 specific disorders.

DSM-I

3 Modern attempts to develop a systematic classification of mental disorders began with DSM-I. Published in 1952 for use in this country, it was developed as an alternative to the mental disorders section of the International Classification of Diseases, Sixth Edition (ICD-6). Although not universally accepted as the official nomenclature throughout this country, it provided, for the first time, a glossary with definitions of categories. It replaced the outdated mental illness section of the Standard Classified Nomenclature of Diseases, the military and Veterans Administration's systems.

DSM-II

In contrast to DSM-I, DSM-II was circulated to 120 psychiatrists with a special interest in the area of diagnosis and was revised based on their criticisms and suggestions. DSM-II, not significantly expanded in size or comprehensiveness, was adopted by the American Psychiatric Association in 1967 and was published and officially accepted throughout this country in 1968. In DSM-II, for the first time, the U.S. classification was based on the mental disorders section of the International Classification of Diseases, Eighth Edition (ICD-8).

DSM-III

In 1974 the American Psychiatric Association (APA) appointed a Task Force on Nomenclature and Statistics to develop DSM-III. DSM-III was prepared by this Task Force, headed by Robert L. Spitzer, M.D., with the aid of 14 advisory committees.

DSM-III, unlike DSM-I and II, was field tested with actual patients. After much controversy and numerous drafts, the third edition of the Diagnostic and Statistical Manual of Mental Disorders, better known as DSM-III, was published in 1980.

DSM-III AND ICD-9

4   DSM-III differs in its content and process of development from DSM-II and from other official classification systems of mental disorders, such as the Ninth Edition of the International Classification of Diseases (ICD-9), and the Clinical Modification (ICD-9-CM) for use in this country.

The International Classification of Diseases is a classification system of many disease entities and is published by the World Health Organization in Geneva for worldwide use. DSM-III was designed with the intent of being a carbon copy or "lift out" of the mental disorders section of ICD-9. However, because of dissatisfaction expressed by organizations representing subspecialties of medicine, this was not accomplished.

Subsequently, the mental disorders section of ICD-9 was modified to allow for greater specificity, in an effort to make it as compatible as possible with DSM-III and acceptable for use in this country. This modification resulted in ICD-9-CM (for clinical modification), which went into effect in this country in January 1979. All DSM-III categories are listed in ICD-9-CM; however, there are some ICD-9-CM categories that are not listed in DSM-III.

DIFFERENCES IN DSM-III

5 DSM-III boasts of many differences or achievements over its predecessors. The following are cited as some of the more significant ones:

- diagnostic criteria
- a redefinition of major conditions, consistent with research findings
- new categories
- a multiaxial system
- a definition of mental disorder

Diagnostic criteria are not vague descriptions, but are specific guidelines designed to assist clinicians in making a diagnosis. They appear at the end of the text for each disorder.

A redefinition of major conditions has occurred as DSM-III sought consistency with research findings. Schizophrenia, for example, is now more narrowly defined.

New categories or modified ones have been included in DSM-III for conditions such as Malingering or Factitious Disorders that previously had no way of being categorized.

A multiaxial system is one of the more prominent achievements of DSM-III and will be discussed later.

A definition of mental disorder was, after several attempts, adopted by the Task Force and various components of the American Psychiatric Association. Every word and comma was carefully examined, resulting in the following definition:

6   In DSM-III each of the mental disorders is conceptualized as a clinically significant behavioral or psychological syndrome or pattern that occurs in an individual and that is typically associated with either a painful symptom (distress) or impairment in one or more important areas of functioning (disability). In addition, there is an inference that there is a behavioral, psychological, or biological dysfunction, and that the disturbance is not only in the relationship between the individual and society. (When the disturbance is *limited* to a conflict between an individual and society, this may represent social deviance which may

or may not be commendable, but is not by itself a mental disorder.)
(DSM-III, p. 6.)

This definition provided concepts useful in making the many decisions that
the Task Force had to face with regard to what conditions to include and how
to define boundaries of the various disorders.

DSM-III takes a phenomenological, descriptive approach rather than an
etiological, theoretical one. It classifies disorders, not individuals.

DSM-III does not assume that disorders have an organic basis or that
they are discrete and discontinuous. It does not assume that groupings of disorders are homogeneous or that disorders are the only appropriate focus of
professional attention.

OBJECTIVES OF DSM-III

There are several objectives of DSM-III. The system attempts to:

- facilitate accurate and clinically relevant diagnosis through detailed
  descriptions and diagnostic criteria.
- enhance the clinician's ability to diagnose, treat, study and communi-
  cate about mental disorders.
- reduce the widespread practice of using a single diagnostic label in
  vastly different ways, and therefore facilitate agreement among clinicians.
- provide a common language for, and enhance communication between, clinicians and research investigators.
- complement, not replace or usurp, the clinician's judgment.

DSM-III does not presume to represent the final solution in the quest for
a more useful and reliable diagnostic system; rather it is a part of an ongoing
process to attempt to classify and understand mental disorders.

Chapter 2

Multiaxial Classification

GENERAL OVERVIEW

DSM-III is the first official multiaxial classification system, described as one that provides for the systematic evaluation of an individual in terms of several variables. In addition to information about the clinical syndrome, the system includes valuable data related to possible etiologic factors, treatment planning and prognosis.

The use of a multiaxial system provides for:

- comprehensiveness of diagnosis and evaluation of mental disorders.
- documentation of multiple classes of information on an individual.
- higher interclinician diagnostic agreement.
- retrieval of statistical and research information.

The idea behind a multiaxial concept is to evaluate and consider all interrelated conditions. For example:

Consider the individual who has an Anxiety Disorder, diabetes and a Personality Disorder. Three different clinicians evaluating this individual might each give three different diagnoses. The internist might focus on the diabetes and ignore the other two disorders, whereas another might focus on the Personality Disorder and ignore the Anxiety Disorder and the diabetes. The multiaxial concept puts these different classes of information on different axes. When attention is directed to each of the three classes of clinical information, all three would be picked up by all of the clinicians.

DSM-III uses five axes in its multiaxial classification scheme. Axes I, II, and III represent the official diagnostic assessment. Axes IV and V, providing information to supplement the official DSM-III diagnoses, are available for use in special clinical and research settings.

The five Axes are:

8

Axis I	• Clinical Syndromes
	• Additional Codes
	• Conditions Not Attributable to a Mental Disorder That Are a Focus of Attention or Treatment
Axis II	• Personality Disorders
	• Specific Developmental Disorders
Axis III	• Physical Disorders and Conditions
Axis IV	• Severity of Psychosocial Stressors
Axis V	• Highest Level of Adaptive Functioning Past Year

AXES I AND II

All clinical syndromes (i.e., Schizophrenia, Affective Disorders and Mental Retardation) plus other conditions that are not mental disorders but are a focus of attention or treatment (i.e., Uncomplicated Bereavement, Parent Child Problems, Malingering), as well as no disorder or condition, are coded on Axis I.

Personality Disorders and Specific Developmental Disorders are coded on Axis II.

This separation was made in an attempt to ensure that Personality Disorders and Specific Developmental Disorders are not overlooked when attention is focused on the more florid symptoms of the Axis I disorders.

These two axes contain the entire DSM-III classification.

AXIS III

This axis permits the clinician to document any physical conditions or disorders that are potentially relevant to the understanding or management of the individual. Any other significant physical findings (e.g., soft neurological signs) may also be listed on Axis III. More than one finding or condition may be listed.

AXIS IV

This axis permits the clinician to identify and evaluate the psychosocial stressors relevant to the assessment and treatment of the individual. The clinician takes note of the number and the severity of life events that are judged significant in the development or exacerbation of the current disorder. DSM-III provides a rating scale as a guide for gauging the severity of the stressors.

AXIS V

This axis permits the clinician to indicate his/her judgment of the peak level of adaptive functioning that an individual has been able to maintain for a period of time during the previous year. A composite of three major areas denotes DSM-III's concept of adaptive functioning: social relations, occupational functioning, and the use of leisure time. A rating scale is provided as a guide for gauging the highest level of adaptive functioning.

SUMMARY

The basic rule with a multiaxial system is that each axis is considered for each individual and the findings, or absence of findings, are so documented. To make it workable, DSM-III restricts the system to a small number of axes that were chosen on the basis of providing information of maximum clinical usefulness in the greatest number of cases.

The following is an example of a multiaxial evaluation:

9

Axis I:	Alcohol Dependence—Episodic
Axis II:	Antisocial Personality
Axis III:	Cirrhosis
Axis IV:	Psychosocial stressors: business failure and marital separation.
	Severity: Severe—5
Axis V:	Highest level of adaptive functioning past year: Poor—5

Due to business failure, the individual has not held a job for more than a few weeks at a time within the past year and, since the marital separation, has been drinking more than usual.

CASE EXAMPLE

The next example is a mystery case or whodunit. This case was presented at the DSM-III workshop in New York City in December 1979 by Robert Spitzer, M.D., and his colleagues.

Axis I:	Cocaine Abuse
Axis II:	Compulsive Personality Disorder and Narcissistic Personality Disorder

Axis III: Gunshot wound
Axis IV: Psychosocial stressors: loss of important case which resulted in severe damage to his career and subsequently a great financial loss.
Severity: Severe—5
Axis V: Highest level adaptive functioning past year: Very Good—2

During the previous year he has stayed on the job and pursued his elusive enemy; he enjoys his work and always gets his man; and spends his leisure time playing the violin. Who is this person?

10   **Answer**—See Answers, Chapter 2.

Section II

Basic Concepts and Use

Chapter 3

Key Concepts in the Use of DSM-III

GENERAL INFORMATION

Previous manuals for DSM-I and DSM-II were barely more than a list of the diagnostic classifications. The designers of DSM-III have included more features.

The DSM-III manual contains the new diagnostic classification, and also addresses the steps in the *process* of diagnosis. There are actually two DSM-III manuals available: the complete 494-page (green) book and the abbreviated 267-page (yellow) pocket edition called the Quick Reference. The complete manual is rather like a textbook, with lengthy sections on the history and development of classification systems, discourses on each major disorder, a glossary, and some appendices on research regarding reliability, and other materials. The Quick Reference eliminates the large areas of text, but contains the vital information on use of the system, the decision trees for differential diagnosis, and the all important diagnostic criteria for the disorders.

DSM-III is not a system that can be used in the clinical setting without the constant employment of one of the manuals. A good plan is to have one complete manual available as a reference text and to have a Quick Reference for everyone's daily use. Another practical idea is to place tabs at those places in the manual and in the Quick Reference that will be referred to frequently (i.e., Axes IV and V, Decision Trees and Major Classifications).

THE DIAGNOSTIC PROCESS

Accurate diagnosis does not begin with the classification system, but with observation of the patient/client. DSM-III cannot supply the skills needed to be

15

a good clinical observer, but it can provide some help even in this first stage of the diagnostic process.

Study of the terms in the glossary can assist in finding the proper standard label for symptoms and features that the patient/client is displaying. It is vital that we use a common and standard technical language in communicating about patients/clients. The terms in the glossary are the vocabulary of this standard technical language. Quite a few of the terms in the glossary are new. Many of the old familiar terms are now defined with more precision and sometimes differently than in the past. It would be a good idea to make sure that one has a complete mastery of the glossary terms before launching into diagnostic classification. The terms aid in discriminating one phenomenon from another; sometimes correct diagnosis will hinge on that proper distinction. The authors of DSM-III have attempted to use the terms in a consistent fashion throughout the manual.

The first step in the diagnostic process consists of accurate recognition of the phenomena confronting the clinician. The second step is proper labeling of those phenomena so that an accurate, succinct portrayal of the features of the presenting disorder can be made. The third step is systematic ruling in or ruling out of alternative disorders which might produce a similar clinical picture; this step is called differential diagnosis.

11   DSM-III provides decision trees to aid in the differential diagnostic process. Beginners with the system may find the decision trees useful; there are eight trees to provide a guide for some of the frequently encountered diagnostic riddles (*Psychiatric Annals*, August 1980, provides trees for the entirety of DSM-III).

Take, for example, the Decision Tree for Mood Disturbance (DSM-III, p. 344). If the clinician had determined that a mood disturbance was present, she/he could start at the top of this decision tree. Going down the tree, a series of simple questions with "yes" or "no" answers guides the clinician on the path to the tentative diagnosis through an orderly process of sorting out the alternatives.

Once a tentative diagnosis is reached, the process of diagnosis is not quite over, but the stage is set for the next step, which includes examination of the diagnostic criteria.

The diagnostician will now look into the manual's section relating to the class of disorders chosen as the tentative diagnosis. All disorders are presented in a uniform format. The manual presents a concise discussion of each class of disorders that includes:

- essential features and a clinical sketch
- features usually associated with the disorder

- typical onset, clinical course, impairment and complications
- specific predisposing factors (if known), prevalence, sex ratio, and familial pattern
- differential diagnostic considerations
- specific diagnostic criteria for the class and all the disorders in it

Each section of the Quick Reference contains only the specific diagnostic criteria for the disorders in that class and brief mention of differential diagnosis.

DIAGNOSTIC CRITERIA AND COMPLETE DIAGNOSIS

For virtually every disorder, DSM-III provides a specific list of features and items of information to be used as a guide to establishing that diagnosis. Diagnostic criteria for any disorder always include a list of features which must be present, along with some other items which must be ruled out before that diagnosis can apply.

12   The diagnostic criteria for Cocaine Intoxication shown in Table 1 are an example of this (DSM-III, pp. 146–147). Different paragraphs deal with different kinds of information. A typical feature is a required number of elements from a list (B & C), and there are always other disorders that must be excluded for this diagnosis to apply (E).

    By following the criteria, the diagnostician can determine if the patient's/client's condition qualifies for the basic diagnosis of the disorder. With many of the disorders, a basic diagnosis is not the complete diagnosis. Many disorders must be further specified as to type, severity, presence of certain associated features, clinical course, or other details. For those disorders requiring more detail for the *complete* diagnosis, the manual and the Quick Reference provide the criteria for those distinctions as well.

13   Diagnostic Criteria for Schizophrenia, Residual Type (DSM-III, pp. 192–193), illustrate that specific criteria are set, not only for the basic disorder, Schizophrenia, but also for each type of Schizophrenia.

14   All DSM-III diagnoses are coded with five digits. For some, the complete five-digit code is provided. For others, such as Schizophrenia, Residual Type, additional determination by the clinician is needed to supply enough information to complete the five-digit code. For all diagnoses needing more information for the fifth digit, the basic code number for the disorders ends with an X, for example 295.6(x). The listing of disorders in the DSM-III classification further reminds the clinician when more information is needed for the complete diagnosis. In addition to the x's, DSM-III leaves a blank space to indicate that further information for the fifth digit must be supplied.

    No diagnosis is complete without enough information to provide for five

TABLE 1
Diagnostic Criteria for Cocaine Intoxication

A. Recent use of cocaine

B. At least two of these symptoms:

 (1) psychomotor agitation
 (2) elation
 (3) grandiosity
 (4) loquacity
 (5) hypervigilance

C. At least two of these symptoms:

 (1) tachycardia
 (2) pupillary dilation
 (3) chills or perspiration
 (4) elevated blood pressure
 (5) nausea and vomiting

D. Maladaptive behavior

E. *Not* due to any other physical or mental disorder

digits. The manual spells out the further criteria for selecting the fifth digit designation. The requirement for this degree of detail in diagnosis is one major reason that a manual (or a Quick Reference) will likely be needed as a guide in diagnosing virtually every case.

HIERARCHICAL PRECEDENCE

The concept of hierarchical precedence applies in DSM-III in two ways:

 (1) Some of the major classes of disorders are so serious that even though the features of a minor disorder are also present, the diagnosis of the major class precludes the use of the minor one.
 (2) Within some classes of disorders, more complex or specific disorders may preclude the additional diagnosis of less complex disorders in the same class.

IMPLICATIONS FOR DIAGNOSTIC INTERVIEWING

Traditionally, diagnostic interviews have tended to be freewheeling and open-ended and the diagnosis was often based on "flavor" or "feel" or some other global impression in the mind of the interviewer. With DSM-III, diagnosis is based on specific criteria for each disorder so that when a given diagnosis is used, we can know quite exactly what is meant because we know that the precise diagnostic criteria have guided the clinician. There is still room for clinical judgment; the criteria are not meant to be rigid inviolable rules, but valuable guides to the clinician.

Since the diagnostic distinctions require specific information, interviewing will have to be designed to secure those details. Interviews will have to be more focused and exploratory and will have to raise questions for the differential diagnostic process.

Diagnosis for DSM-III cannot be based on a "mental status" type of interview only; the longitudinal story as well as the cross-sectional exam will be required. A number of disorders are indistinguishable on cross-section, and are defined by the difference in the longitudinal course.

Some diagnostic distinctions depend on the connection, or lack of it, between life events and the occurrence of the disorder. Consequently, the interviewer has to search for possible connections between the onset of the patient's symptoms and stressors in the past, present, or looming in the future.

Chapter 4

Survey of the
Major Classifications

GENERAL INFORMATION

This chapter provides a quick tour through all the categories included in DSM-III for Axes I and II. It includes *all* the designated categories of mental disorders as well as a category for some related conditions that are discussed in DSM-III but are not called mental disorders.

The more than 200 distinguishable disorders and conditions included in DSM-III have been grouped in a logical and consistent manner. The purpose of this survey is to acquaint participants/readers with the concepts involved in this systematic grouping, and to highlight some of the boundary definitions that help to separate one class of disorders from another.

Practically speaking, there are 18 classes or groups of conditions in DSM-III. (See DSM-III, pp. 15–19.)

15

(1) Disorders Usually First Evident in Infancy, Childhood, or Adolescence

(2) Substance Use Disorders

(3) Organic Mental Disorders

(4) Schizophrenic Disorders

(5) Psychotic Disorders Not Elsewhere Classified

(6) Paranoid Disorders

(7) Affective Disorders

(8) Anxiety Disorders

(9) Dissociative Disorders

(10) Somatoform Disorders

(11) Factitious Disorders
(12) Psychosexual Disorders
(13) Disorders of Impulse Control Not Elsewhere Classified
(14) Adjustment Disorders
(15) Psychological Factors Affecting Physical Condition
(16) V Codes for Conditions Not Attributable to a Mental Disorder
(17) Personality Disorders
(18) Specific Developmental Disorders

This survey does not present the classifications in precisely the same order as the sequences in DSM-III but is arranged to highlight some of the boundary definitions setting off one class of disorders from another. There is no simple, perfect flow in this sequence, but, in general, the classification begins with disorders arising in early years, then disorders with some organic element, then major (psychotic) disorders, followed by more and more minor classes of disorders and the two Axis II disorders. Sixteen of these classes (#1 through #16) are recorded on Axis I; only two (#17 and #18) are recorded on Axis II.

AXIS I

Disorders Usually First Evident in Infancy, Childhood, or Adolescence
This is the classification for disorders which are usually first evident in the early years (infancy, childhood, or adolescence). These are not the only disorders that might be seen during those years, but they are the ones seen most frequently.

This class is not an exclusive subset for children. *All* of DSM-III applies to children as well as adults. Of course, it is a good idea to check this section first for children and the other sections first for adults. But children can have diagnoses from other sections and adults can have diagnoses from this section. This section merely contains some disorders which *typically* arise in the early years.

If a youngster meets the criteria for a disorder in another class, then that diagnosis would be made. Gender Disorders and Schizophrenia are examples of disorders listed elsewhere that certainly can apply to children or adolescents.

Even though the term "adolescence" appears in the title, some of these disorders quite typically arise in the college years (i.e., Identity Disorder).

Older adults may be given some of these diagnoses:

- If the condition arose in early years and has now persisted well into adulthood, and no other diagnosis takes precedence, a diagnosis from this classification may be made. For example, Infantile Autism or Mental Retardation would still apply as the diagnosis even if the individual has aged to 35 (if manifestations of the disorder are still evident).
- Sometimes the condition simply first appears well into adulthood. For example, Anorexia Nervosa usually begins earlier, but could make its first appearance in someone's early 30s.

This very large class is divided into five realms: intellectual, behavioral, emotional, physical, and developmental.

Substance Use Disorders
The word "substance" in the title of this class refers to alcohol, drugs, or tobacco, and its abnormal consumption. This diagnosis is of a pattern of *behavior*—the maladaptive use of some substance. Simple use or consumption of a substance does not constitute a disorder; an *abnormal* pattern of use must be established and contrasted with simple recreational use or legitimate medical use.

Separate diagnoses are required for the abnormal *use* of the substance and for any conditions that may be *consequences* of the Substance Use Disorder on the central nervous system. Those disorders that may be consequences of the Substance Use Disorder are in the class of Organic Mental Disorders. The reason for requiring both diagnoses is that the focus in treatment will shift between managing the abnormal consumption itself and managing the effects of that consumption (abnormal drinking goes in this class, drunkenness goes under Organic Mental Disorders).

Organic Mental Disorders
All of these disorders are caused by transient or permanent dysfunction of brain tissue; dysfunction may be caused by either chemical effects or disease processes.

Precise diagnosis of these disorders depends on evidence (history, physical, lab) to confirm the organicity, and possibly the etiology, but often the clinician can be confident of the organic basis even before conclusive evidence is at hand.

There is no longer the "acute" vs "chronic brain syndrome" of DSM-I; nor is there the "psychotic" vs "non-psychotic organic brain syndrome" of DSM-II. Instead, there are a number of clinicially distinct syndromes to identify. Once the *syndrome* is identified, the disorder is classified according to the causative process.

Disorders with an organic basis always take precedence over other diagnoses that might present exactly the same clinical picture. For example, if a person developed a clinical picture of a paranoid delusional state due to the effects of amphetamines, the diagnosis *must* be that of an Organic Mental Disorder.

Schizophrenic Disorders

There have been big changes in this class of disorders. Research findings have been used to tighten the diagnostic criteria and definition of Schizophrenia.

The basic disorder requires:

- deterioration from a previously accomplished level of functioning (longitudinal);
- pervasive disruption in a whole range of areas of mental functioning (cross-sectional . . . "mental status") (examination of symptoms).

There has to be florid psychosis (e.g., delusions, hallucinations, catatonic features, or marked disruption of thought processes) during an active phase of the illness.

If this picture is present but is the outgrowth of an Organic Mental Disorder, the organic diagnosis prevails. If this picture is present as the outgrowth of a severe mood disturbance, the diagnosis of Affective Disorder prevails.

The total continuous period of illness (continual uninterrupted presence of some symptoms, not just psychotic symptoms) must have lasted for at least six months. Acute psychotic breaks must be diagnosed as another condition in the class of Psychotic Disorders Not Elsewhere Classified.

There is no nonpsychotic type. Individuals diagnosed as having Schizophrenia must have been psychotic at some point. When one encounters what once was called "simple schizophrenia," "latent schizophrenia," or "pseudoneurotic schizophrenia," one now has to consider the class of Personality Disorders.

Psychotic Disorders Not Elsewhere Classified

There are four Psychotic Disorders that are not classified elsewhere: Brief Reactive Psychosis, Schizophreniform Disorder, Schizoaffective Disorder, and Atypical Psychosis.

Brief Reactive Psychosis and Schizophreniform Disorder are clinically indistinguishable from Schizophrenia. It is the longitudinal story that establishes the difference. Brief Reactive Psychosis is what was once unofficially called "hysterical psychosis" or "three-day schizophrenia." Schizophreniform Disorder is what was once called "acute schizophrenic episode." The picture can be exactly the same as Schizophrenia, but without continuous symptoms for a full six months. Schizoaffective Disorder and Atypical Psychosis are used when no clear distinction can be made, but a Psychotic Disorder is recognized.

Paranoid Disorders
Paranoid Disorders can best be understood in contrast to Schizophrenia and Psychotic Disorders Not Elsewhere Classified. Schizophrenia and similar disorders are more pervasively disruptive and incapacitating, with symptoms involving many areas of mental functioning.

In the Paranoid Disorders, there is rarely more than a set of delusions in an otherwise generally intact individual; there is rarely impairment in intellect or daily occupational functioning. There are no prominent hallucinations. Aside from the delusions, the individual has good reality-testing, and the delusions do not have the bizarre, patently absurd characteristics of schizophrenic ones.

The delusions in Paranoid Disorders are of two kinds:

(1) Persecutory ("people out to get me")
(2) Jealous (delusion of betrayal)

Affective Disorders
Affective Disorders involve a primary disturbance in *mood*. Mood is a pervasive emotion and there can eventually be distortions in thinking and behavior as a result of the disturbance.

Persons with Major Affective Disorders may develop delusions or hallucinations as the condition intensifies. They may eventually develop psychotic features that are not congruent with the mood, and the diagnosis will still apply since the mood disturbance itself was the primary and originating factor. (The mood disturbance must not have been preceded by characteristic schizophrenic symptoms.)

This boundary definition makes Affective Disorders much broader, and Schizophrenic Disorders somewhat narrower, than in the past.

The basic mood derangements are manic syndromes (elations) or depressive syndromes. The exact designation of each Affective Disorder is dependent on certain additional patterns and features such as degree of severity, duration, and pattern of mood over time.

Any affective syndrome due to an organic basis requires an organic diagnosis rather than one of Affective Disorder.

Anxiety Disorders

The class of Anxiety Disorders is a new grouping that is largely the outgrowth of research findings. It promises to be a practical and clinically useful classification.

In all these disorders, anxiety is actually a prominent part of the clinical picture. It may be experienced spontaneously as panic, generalized anxiety, or traumatic flashbacks. It may be experienced directly if the person resists phobic, obsessive, or compulsive symptoms.

One would not make a diagnosis of Anxiety Disorder in the face of a more severe disorder that could be responsible for the Anxiety Disorder features. Individuals with Schizophrenia or Affective Disorders may have all the symptoms of an Anxiety Disorder without requiring a separate diagnosis.

Dissociative Disorders

This is a traditional grouping of disorders which all feature dissociation: sudden, temporary alteration in a usually intact consciousness, identity, or motor behavior. Some part of these complex functions goes along on its own, detached and not incorporated with the rest of the individual's experience.

In amnesia, some important events are lost from an otherwise intact memory. In a fugue, a person travels a considerable distance and sets up a new life with no recall of his previous life. In multiple personality, one's customary identity is lost while another identity takes over and dominates the individual's existence. Each personality is distinct and relatively complete. Depersonalization Disorder involves a significant degree of experiences such as disembodiment, and other uncanny sensations.

Somatoform Disorders

The class of Somatoform Disorders deals with the presentation of physical complaints, or what appear to be physical symptoms, that have no organic basis.

However, the absence of an organic basis and the impression of causative psychological factors does not in itself make the distinction that sets the boundary for these disorders. That distinction is based on controllability of the symptoms. To qualify as a Somatoform Disorder, the symptoms must be judged *not to be under voluntary control*. Should the person be able to turn the physical symptoms off and on deliberately, the diagnosis would be a Factitious Disorder or Malingering, which is classified as a Condition Not Attributable to a Mental Disorder.

Factitious Disorders

These cases may also present with what appear to be physical symptoms that have no genuine organic basis. But in this case, the person is deliberately turning the symptom on or off; it is under voluntary control (unlike a Somatoform Disorder).

What distinguishes Factitious Disorders from outright Malingering is that individuals with Factitious Disorders have no goal other than becoming, or continuing to be, a patient. Some Factitious Disorders involve the fabrication of psychological symptoms such as faking a portrayal of psychosis or dementia to secure a chance to be a patient. Someone who would fake such symptoms to achieve other goals, such as monetary gain or evasion of prosecution, would be demonstrating Malingering.

Psychosexual Disorders

This class is all inclusive, applying to all sexual disorders that do not have an organic basis (children and adults). It covers a range from the mild and mundane to the severe and bizarre.

Gender Identity Disorders involve a powerful wish to be the opposite sex. Paraphilias involve abnormal dependence on abnormal objects or situations to achieve sexual arousal. Psychosexual Dysfunctions are typed by the phase in the sexual response cycle in which they occur: desire, excitement, or orgasm.

Since "ego-syntonic homosexuality" is no longer officially considered a mental disorder, only ego-dystonic homosexuality would be classified here under Other Psychosexual Disorders.

Disorders of Impulse Control Not Elsewhere Classified

These impulsive behaviors are all ego-syntonic and voluntary. They are not compulsions, nor are they dissociative or psychotic phenomena.

Each involves some action that could harm the individual himself, or others, while relieving a buildup of tension. There is either pleasure or a sense of release in the act, but often a strong remorse afterwards.

Impulsive behavior that is a manifestation of other disorders, such as Attention Deficit Disorder, would not require this diagnosis. If the impulsive behavior cannot be explained as a part of some other condition, then this class should be considered.

Adjustment Disorders
These are relatively minor disorders. Possible diagnoses from other classes should be considered and ruled out before considering this class. If the criteria for one of the major classes (such as Anxiety Disorder, Affective Disorder, a Psychotic Disorder) are met, then that diagnosis takes precedence.

The Adjustment Disorders require:

- the occurrence of a life event, without which no disorder would exist;
- the individual engages in a maladaptive response to the life event, producing the current symptoms;
- the person can be expected to return to normal when the psychosocial stressor is gone. The particular stressors should be listed and rated on Axis IV.

Psychological Factors Affecting Physical Condition
This diagnosis indicates, first of all, that there is a physical condition that warrants being recorded on Axis III. It also indicates that the physical condition appears to be aggravated in some way by psychological factors. The physical condition may show greater severity of symptoms, increased frequency of attacks, or more difficulty in management. For example:

(1) Asthma attacks occur with greater frequency and severity because of the apprehension of final exams.

(2) Obesity is unmanageable since the person is too anxious to follow a diet.

V Codes for Conditions Not Attributable to a Mental Disorder That Are a Focus of Attention or Treatment
This is *not* a term that is meant to indicate that these conditions are not as genuine or legitimate as the official disorders; rather, it indicates that the definition of "mental disorder" is not met.

Individuals with these conditions might very justifiably seek mental health care. Services such as marital counseling, rape counseling, and educational programs would find that this class is often used.

DSM-III lists some of the V Codes that are found in ICD-9-CM (i.e., Child Abuse, Malingering, and Borderline Intellectual Functioning). ICD-9-CM has a much more extensive listing of V Codes for conditions not attributable to a mental disorder that, nevertheless, might be the focus of evaluation, attention, or treatment.

AXIS II

Personality Disorders and Specific Developmental Disorders are the only classes that are noted on Axis II.

Personality Disorders

Personality Disorders are composed of maladaptive, pervasive personality traits exhibited so extremely and in such a wide range of contexts that subjective distress and/or impaired functioning results. These patterns of traits are generally recognizable by adolescence or even earlier and persist through adult life. In *some* children and adolescents, these patterns are set clearly and enduringly enough that these diagnoses can be used.

DSM-III is not categorizing personality type or profile, but disorders in personality. A person has only one personality but can display more than one Personality Disorder.

Specific Developmental Disorders

These disorders are placed on Axis II, in part, to assure that they will not be overlooked. They are found most commonly in youngsters but can occasionally be found in adults. These disorders are listed in a special box as part of Disorders Usually First Evident in Infancy, Childhood, or Adolescence, but they are treated as a class by themselves.

Previously called "learning disabilities," these disorders involve a substantial delay in acquiring or learning some specific function. The delay must not be accounted for as simply part of a person's Axis I disorder that would include an overall general delay in development (for example, Mental Retardation or Infantile Autism).

MAJOR DIFFERENCES BETWEEN DSM-II AND DSM-III

DSM-II made only sweeping distinctions between Organic Mental Disorders as psychotic or nonpsychotic. Organic Mental Disorders are now defined as precise clinical syndromes.

Schizophrenia is now a much narrower concept, with the nonpsychotic and the brief psychotic forms categorized elsewhere. Schizophrenia may now represent a more consistent clinical entity, a major disabling disorder with a tendency to recur and cause severe functional impairment.

All primary disorders of mood are now grouped together as Affective Disorders rather than scattered through various sections. Affective Disorders have a somewhat broader range, including some cases that would have been called Schizophrenia in the past.

Adjustment Disorders are now limited to minor maladjustments that do not reach the magnitude of the major disorders.

In DSM-II, there was a "psychophysiologic disorders" section; disorders listed there had authentic physical signs and were stated to be of psychogenic origin. DSM-III authors chose to emphasize the *interplay* between physical and emotional factors.

The issue of physical-appearing symptoms which have no genuine organic basis has been sorted out by distinguishing between Somatoform Disorders, Factitious Disorders, and Malingering.

DSM-III is atheoretical; it is "phenomenologically descriptive." The traditional term "neurosis" implied an etiological concept, presumably common to some diverse disorders for most of which there is considerable evidence for alternative theories of causation. Most disorders in the DSM-II "neurosis" section are now grouped in other ways, along with other disorders with phenomenological similarity.

Previously, a number of recognizable clinical conditions were not listed in DSM-II. Now virtually all the universally recognized conditions are listed, with diagnostic criteria for each.

Rather than feeling forced artificially toward "the one right diagnosis," the clinician using DSM-III's multiaxial system can record the true complexity and/or ambiguity of the clinical situation.

Chapter 5

Use of Axes I and II

AXIS I AND AXIS II TOGETHER
As previously indicated, all disorders and conditions listed in DSM-III are recorded on Axis I, except for Personality Disorders and Specific Developmental Disorders, which are recorded on Axis II.

16   The diagnostician must complete each axis by recording a diagnosis or by recording that no disorder exists on that axis. In some cases an individual will have a disorder on both axes. In others there may be a disorder on Axis I with no disorder on Axis II. Or it can be the other way around.

EXAMPLES:

Axis I: Opioid Abuse, Episodic
Axis II: Antisocial Personality Disorder

Axis I: Major Depression, Recurrent
Axis II: No Disorder

Axis I: No Disorder
Axis II: Dependent Personality Disorder

MULTIPLE DIAGNOSES
DSM-III encourages multiple diagnoses on a single axis when needed to define the current conditions. An individual may have one, two, or more disorders on a single axis. When there is more than one disorder to list, first write the condition taking priority for clinical attention.

17   The following example illustrates a man seen in an emergency room for

drunkenness. He is known to have a full depressive syndrome which at the moment is not the urgent focus of clinical management.

EXAMPLE:

> **Axis I:**   Alcohol Intoxication
> Major Depression, Single Episode

18   Another individual with a Compulsive Personality Disorder also has a Paranoid Personality Disorder. (In addition to being rigid, perfectionistic and demanding, he is irascible, alienating and constantly blames everyone else.)

EXAMPLE:

> **Axis II:**   Compulsive Personality Disorder
> Paranoid Personality Disorder

19   A person may have multiple diagnoses on *both* Axis I *and* Axis II, as this example illustrates.

EXAMPLE:

> **Axis I:**   Alcohol Withdrawal
> Alcohol Dependence, Continuous
>
> **Axis II:**   Dependent Personality Disorder
> Histrionic Personality Disorder

LEVELS OF DIAGNOSTIC CERTAINTY
There are some clinical situations where the diagnosis can be known with certainty, but with others there is not enough information to precisely identify a disorder.

DSM-III provides a way for the diagnostician to identify the degree of certainty to which there is, or is not, a disorder, and, if a disorder is present, what it is.

Diagnosis Deferred is used when there is inadequate information to reach a conclusion as to whether or not the person has a disorder on Axis I or Axis II.

No Disorder is used to indicate that the clinician searched for a disorder on one or the other axis and has drawn a clear conclusion that there is no disorder present. "No Disorder" is a positive and conclusive statement.

Unspecified Mental Disorder (nonpsychotic) is used on Axis I when the clinician is able to recognize that the person definitely has some disorder or condition, but can only determine that it is not a psychotic disorder.

Atypical Psychosis is used on Axis I when a clinician recognizes the presence of a psychotic disorder that does not meet the criteria for a specific mental disorder.

Atypical (Class of the Disorder That Is Recognized) Disorder is used when the clinician recognizes what general class or subclass the diagnosis belongs in, but is unable to be exactly sure where *within* the class this condition belongs. For example, if a man had nearly constant bouts of anxiety and tension, an Anxiety Disorder might be recognized, but it might not be possible to find a satisfying niche within the class for an exact fit, so the term "Atypical Anxiety Disorder" would be used to show that it is in that ballpark.

20   **Provisional** is used when the clinician has been able to settle on the precise diagnosis, but has some doubts about it. For example, by indicating "(Provisional)" after Brief Reactive Psychosis, the clinician is able to express that this could turn out to have been a drug-induced episode.

PREMORBID PERSONALITY AND PERSONALITY TRAITS (AXIS II)

21   **Premorbid** is used whenever an Axis I disorder obscures someone's usual personality features, but it is known that the person's lifelong character pattern has included a Personality Disorder. The term "(Premorbid)" is indicated after the Axis II diagnosis. For example, Axis II: Histrionic Personality Disorder (Premorbid).

Sometimes a person clearly shows distinct personality traits, but not to a sufficient extent to qualify for an actual Personality Disorder. Because awareness of those traits might influence understanding and management of the case, it is valuable to recognize them on the multiaxial scheme. For example, a person who demonstrates an exaggerated emotional expressiveness and a tendency to overreact to rather insignificant events in his/her life, but who does not meet any of the other criteria for a Histrionic Personality Disorder, would not be given a Personality Disorder diagnosis. In this case, Histrionic Personality traits could be noted on Axis II.

If only traits are recorded on Axis II, no disorder will ultimately be coded for statistical purposes.

PRINCIPAL DIAGNOSIS
Unless otherwise stated, the principal diagnosis, the condition chiefly responsible for initiating the evaluation or care, will be presumed to be the first condition listed on Axis I.

Whenever an Axis II disorder is the condition chiefly under consideration, the Axis II disorder should be designated as the principal diagnosis.

For example, in this case a person with a dormant drinking problem is enrolled in a group therapy program aimed at characterological problems:

Axis I: Alcohol Abuse, Episodic, In Remission

Axis II: Dependent Personality Disorder (Principal Diagnosis)

Unless the Axis II disorder is designated as the principal diagnosis, it is assumed to be on Axis I.

Chapter 6

Use of Axis III

GENERAL INFORMATION
DSM-III's multiaxial framework provides a comprehensive look at the individual, with a different kind of information on each axis.

Axis III is the location for recording all known, significant medical and physical conditions. This approach should assure that as clinicians focus on mental problems, they don't fail to acknowledge some physical condition important in understanding or managing the case. Every conceivable physical condition is listed and coded in ICD-9-CM, including physical conditions with external causes such as injuries, toxic reactions, etc.

RELATION OF AXIS III TO AXES I AND II
22 Sometimes the physical condition is important to note because it is etiologic to the mental disorder, such as Axis I: Organic Affective Syndrome, Axis III: Huntington's Chorea. Another example would be liver failure on Axis III responsible for delirium on Axis I.

23 Quite commonly, the Axis III disorder is not etiologic, but is related to Axis I. For example, an overly dependent person may have consumed alcohol in such a maladaptive way that alcoholic gastritis resulted. The diagnoses would be recorded as follows:

> Axis I: Alcohol Dependence, Continuous
> Axis II: Dependent Personality Disorder
> Axis III: Alcoholic Gastritis

Some of the complex interactions are elucidated by the multiaxial scheme.

Often, the physical condition is neither etiologic nor interrelated, but is nonetheless important to note for the overall understanding and management of the case. Diabetes, for example, should be noted even though unrelated to the mental disorder.

Quite often, there will be no known significant physical condition; this is indicated by writing "None known" for Axis III.

24   Sometimes the individual's reason for seeking treatment is an injury that was accidentally or purposefully inflicted by self or others (i.e., suicide, human stampede, poisoning). These conditions, found in ICD-9-CM, are given E Codes and may be recorded on Axis III.

Chapter 7

Use of Axis IV

GENERAL OVERVIEW

Axis IV, considered optional by the American Psychiatric Association, provides for a rating of the overall severity of stressors that are judged to have contributed to the development or exacerbation of the current disorder.

The judgment of the severity of the psychosocial stressors takes into account:

25

- the amount of change in the individual's life caused by the stressor;
- the degree to which the stressor or event is desired;
- the degree to which the event is under the individual's control;
- the number of stressors.

The rating of the severity of the stressors is based on the clinician's assessment of the stress that an "average" person would experience under similar circumstances. "Average" refers to a person with similar sociocultural values. In addition, the rating is based on the severity of the stressor itself, not on the vulnerability of the individual. For example, a 40-year-old individual who has never been on a vacation in his life may experience this as a major event; however, on the continuum of stressors, relative to divorce or death, this vacation is only a minimal or mild stressor.

In determining the psychosocial stressors that are contributing to the current disorder, it is necessary to assess stressors within one year prior to the onset. In some cases, such as Post-traumatic Stress Disorder, the stressor will have occurred more than one year prior to the onset of symptoms. Also, in some instances the stressor is the anticipation of a future event, for instance, knowledge that one will soon graduate from college and apply for a job.

TYPES OF PSYCHOSOCIAL STRESSORS

Psychosocial stressors are any situations or events that produce some change in an individual's life requiring that he/she adapt or cope with the resultant stress.

Stressors may also be an outgrowth of a mental disorder. For example, in the case of an individual with the diagnosis of Alcohol Abuse, marital problems may result from excessive drinking. The marital problems may then further contribute to and exacerbate the mental disorder of Alcohol Abuse.

26   Axis IV applies to adults and children and adolescents.

The types of psychosocial stressors that may be considered include the following:

27
- conjugal (marital or nonmarital): divorce, discord, engagement
- parenting: friction with child
- other interpersonal: illness of friend, discord with friend or boss
- occupational: retirement, job change, unemployment, school problems
- living circumstances: change in residence, burglary
- financial: bank loan, bankruptcy, inheritance
- legal: lawsuit, jail
- developmental: menopause, turning 40, puberty
- physical illness or injury: accident, surgery
- family factors (children and adolescents): overtly hostile relationship between parents, parental intrusiveness
- other: natural disaster, rape

Other examples of stressors that may be considered for children and adolescents are:

28
- foster placement
- physical or mental abuse or neglect
- physical or mental disturbance in family member
- loss of a nuclear family member

RATING THE SEVERITY OF THE STRESSORS

29   The rating for the severity of the psychosocial stressors is on a scale from 1 (none) to 7 (catastrophic), as indicated in Table 2. When determining the rating, only the stressors that have exacerbated or contributed to the onset of the mental disorder should be taken into consideration. There may be one or more stressors that are judged to be etiologically significant. The rating should reflect the summed effect of all the psychosocial stressors.

TABLE 2
Severity of Psychosocial Stressors

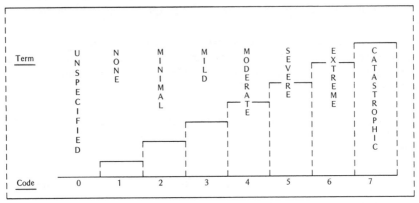

Since Axis IV is a new component of the diagnostic system, it is not as advanced or refined in its development as the other axes. The determination of the rating will depend on the best judgment of the clinician or treatment team.

Guidelines for determining the ratings for both adults and children or adolescents are found in the DSM-III manual (p. 27) and in Table 3. In addition, the research by Holmes and Rahe (1967) on life event experiences provides a guide to help determine the relative severity of different stressors.

CASE VIGNETTE

Susan, 15 years old, is an only child living with her mother and father. She has always done fairly well in school, making C's and B's, and has several friends in her neighborhood. She has not, however, formed any close friends in school, and has no hobbies or interests other than school.

Nine months ago, Susan's maternal grandmother, who had been living with the family for the past three years, died. Three months after the death of the grandmother, the family moved to a different neighborhood in the same city.

Shortly after the move, Susan began to resist going to school. About once or twice a week she would come home early because she felt sick. The results of a parent-teacher meeting indicated that Susan's grades have dropped one letter grade.

Discussion Guide

The severity of the psychosocial stressors is judged to be severe because of the death of the grandmother coupled with a change in residence.

30   **Answer**—See Answers, Chapter 7, a.

CASE VIGNETTE

Cindy is a 28-year-old speech therapist working in a school district's special education division. For all of her adult life she has been bothered by low-

TABLE 3

Use of Axis IV: Rating Examples of Psychosocial Stressors*

Code	Term	Adult Example	Child or Adolescent Example
1	None	None Apparent.	None Apparent.
2	Minimal	Small bank loan; minor violation of the law.	Vacation with family.
3	Mild	Change in residence; change in working hours or conditions.	New school year; change in day care center; insufficient parental control.
4	Moderate	Death of close friend; new career; sexual difficulties.	Change to new school; birth of a sibling; illness of close relative.
5	Severe	Personal injury or illness; marriage; marital separation; major financial loss; fired from job.	Divorce of parents; hospitalization; major illness in family member; arrest; harsh and persistent parental discipline.
6	Fxtreme	Divorce; death of a spouse or child; jail term.	Death of parent or sibling; physical or sexual abuse; severe injury or illness resulting in paralysis or loss of a limb.
7	Catastrophic	Devastating natural disaster; multiple family deaths; concentration camp experience.	Multiple family deaths.
0	Unspecified	No information or not applicable.	No information or not applicable.

*These examples represent relative severity of stressors, not their cumulative effect.

grade depressive symptoms. She has stretches of normal moods for a few days at a time, but they always subside into the gloomy mood that has become a way of life for her. Nonetheless, she has always managed to function in a manner that gives co-workers no clue that she is depressed.

Two months ago the elderly and benevolent woman supervising Cindy's department retired and she was replaced by a vigorous 30-year-old man with an entirely different approach to supervision. He immediately instituted rigid procedures and generated a cold, strictly business atmosphere. Cindy now finds that her mood has worsened. She can no longer disguise the fact from her co-workers and she is afraid that the new supervisor will notice her depressed condition and that she may get a poor performance rating.

Discussion Guide
The only notable stressor is the change in boss and work environment, thus the severity of psychosocial stressors is judged to be mild. The stressor exacerbated the depression in this case. The mild rating represents what an average person would experience in this case, even though Cindy's perception of this stressor and reaction was more than "mild."

31   **Answer**—See Answers, Chapter 7, b.

Chapter 8

Use of Axis V

GENERAL OVERVIEW

Axis V provides for a rating of the highest level of adaptive functioning maintained for at least a few months during the past year. Like Axis IV, the use of Axis V is considered to be optional by the American Psychiatric Association.

32   Adaptive function, as conceptualized in the DSM-III, is a composite of three areas: social relations, occupational functioning, and leisure time.

AREAS OF ADAPTIVE FUNCTIONING

Social relations refers to all interpersonal relations but with particular emphasis placed on friends and family. The breadth and quality of relationships are also taken into consideration.

      Occupational functioning refers to the amount, complexity, and the quality of the work accomplished as a worker, student, or homemaker.

      Leisure time includes the range and depth of involvement in recreational activities or hobbies.

RATING THE LEVEL OF ADAPTIVE FUNCTIONING

33 The rating of adaptive functioning applies to adults as well as children and adolescents and is based on a determination of the highest level of functioning which was sustained for at least a few months during the past year.

34   The rating scale for the highest level of adaptive functioning during the past year is on a continuum from 1 (superior) to 7 (grossly impaired), as indicated in Table 4.

      While the rating takes into account social relations, occupational func-

TABLE 4
Levels of Adaptive Functioning

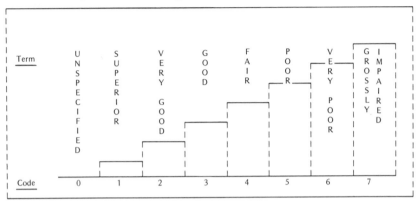

tioning, and use of leisure time, greater weight should be given to social relations because of its greater prognostic significance.

The rating of Superior—1 should be used only when there is no subjective discomfort associated with high occupational functioning.

The assessment of the use of leisure time should affect the overall rating only when occupational opportunities are limited or there is no significant impairment in social relations and occupational functioning.

The rating should reflect the individual's highest level of functioning even if special circumstances, such as a halfway house or other treatment, were necessary to sustain the level.

Guidelines or examples for determining the rating for various levels of adaptive functioning are provided in DSM-III (pp. 29 & 30) and in Table 5. In addition, the work done by Newman and Rinkus (1978) provides further guidelines for differentiating between the levels of functioning.

CASE VIGNETTE

Mark is a 43-year-old married assembly line worker with two children. He has few friends outside the family and basically keeps to himself. He enjoys fishing and will take his sons with him once or twice a month. Mark's wife encourages him to attend church with her; however, he refuses and they have had repeated fights in the past year over his refusal.

Mark was employed by General Motors for the past 10 years and his performance evaluations indicated that he was an average worker with a good

TABLE 5
Use of Axis V: Rating Scale and Examples for Use of Axis V

Level	Adult Example	Child or Adolescent Example
1 SUPERIOR—Unusually effective functioning in social relations, occupational functioning, and use of leisure time. No distress associated with occupational functioning.	A single parent functions extremely well on the job, takes excellent care of the children, has several close friends, and pursues an interest in music.	A 12-year-old gets excellent grades in school, has numerous friends, and excels in soccer and swimming.
2 VERY GOOD—Better than average functioning in social relations, occupational functioning, and use of leisure time.	A single parent does all of the above but complains of feeling stressed on the job.	A 12-year-old does all of the above but complains of some distress in keeping up with both school and sports.
3 GOOD—No more than slight impairment in either social or occupational functioning.	A single parent functions well on the job, takes excellent care of the children, has several close friends, but has no leisure interests or pursuits.	A 12-year-old participates in school activities and sports, has numerous friends, but has some difficulty maintaining a C average in school.
4 FAIR—Moderate impairment in either social relations or occupational functioning, or some impairment in both.	A single parent has difficulty carrying through with job assignments and has several acquaintances, but no close friends.	A 12-year-old gets average grades in school, has only one friend, and does not participate in any social activities.
5 POOR—Marked impairment in either social relations or occupational functioning, or moderate impairment in both.	A single parent has difficulty keeping a job for more than a few weeks.	A 12-year-old has no friends and is getting failing grades in two subjects at school.
6 VERY POOR—Marked impairment in both social relations and occupational functioning.	A single parent has difficulty keeping a job for more than a few weeks, has no close friends or acquaintances, and has frequent angry outbursts with neighbors and family.	A 12-year-old has no friends and is failing in all subjects at school.
7 GROSSLY IMPAIRED—Gross impairment in virtually all areas of functioning.	A single parent is unable to care for the home or children, does not attend to personal hygiene, and is usually incoherent.	A 12-year-old is unable to attend school, is unable to attend to personal hygiene, and refuses to talk to family or friends.
O UNSPECIFIED	No information.	No information.

work attendance. Thirteen months ago Mark was laid off from his job, presumably because of fluctuations in the economy. He reported feeling discouraged about the layoff and had difficulty finding similar work. Six months ago he finally took a job making hospital beds to help support the family, but he feels dissatisfied with this type of job.

In the past month Mark has become increasingly withdrawn. He no longer takes the children fishing, and he has mentioned separating from his wife.

Discussion Guide
Mark is not functioning at his potential occupational level and has few friends or social contacts outside his family. He does, however, pursue his hobby, fishing, with his sons. Thus Mark's highest level of adaptive functioning for at least a few months during the past year is considered to be fair.

35   **Answer**—See Answers, Chapter 8, a.

CASE VIGNETTE
Roger is a nine-year-old boy with Down's Syndrome. He has for the past three years attended a school for the retarded. His teachers reported that he was an average student who performed assigned tasks appropriately, needing additional assistance on occasion. He had numerous friends at school, got along well with other children, and had been a bat boy for his 21-year-old brother's neighborhood softball team.

However, ten months ago, Roger's parents separated and since then he has been living with his mother, visiting his father only once or twice during the separation. Four months ago Roger's older brother married and moved out of the house. In addition, Roger's teacher retired, and he has had a new teacher for the past six months.

During the past two months Roger has become physically violent at school. He gets into numerous fights with his classmates and has on two occasions been caught purse-snatching from teachers. His school performance has dropped off considerably; however, it is still considered in the adequate range.

Discussion Guide
For all but the last two months, Roger has functioned adequately at school and has numerous friends. In addition, he enjoys leisure activities with his

family. Thus Roger's highest level of adaptive functioning during the past year is considered to be good.

36   **Answer**—See Answers, Chapter 8, b.

Section III

Review of Major Classifications

Chapter 9

Disorders Usually First Evident in Infancy, Childhood, or Adolescence

GENERAL OVERVIEW

This classification describes disorders that usually begin or become evident in infancy, childhood, or adolescence.

In diagnosing Disorders Usually First Evident in Infancy, Childhood, or Adolescence, clinicians should have a basic knowledge of normal development in order to be able to distinguish between normal temperamental age variations and full clinical syndromes.

This class of disorders should be reviewed first when assessing an infant, child, or adolescent. However, disorders from other sections should be used if the child or adolescent demonstrates symptoms that meet the diagnostic criteria of any of the Substance Use Disorders, Schizophrenic Disorders, Anxiety Disorders, etc.

DSM-III does not set rigid or arbitrary age boundaries for infancy, childhood, or adolescence. Some disorders *do* mention a specific age in the diagnostic criteria and these should be followed. However, all diagnostic criteria should be considered for individuals of any age.

Although disorders in this section *usually* occur in infancy, childhood, or adolescence, they can develop in early or later adulthood (e.g., Anorexia Nervosa). Adults can manifest conditions in this section that have persisted into adulthood (e.g., Attention Deficit Disorder, Residual Type). In these cases diagnoses from this section should be used for adults.

The disorders in this section can be grouped into five categories based on the area of functioning that seems to be central to the disturbance. These categories are:

37   (1) Intellectual
                  Mental Retardation

            (2) Behavioral
                  Attention Deficit Disorder
                  Conduct Disorder

            (3) Emotional
                  Anxiety Disorders of Childhood or Adolescence
                  Other Disorders of Infancy, Childhood, or Adolescence

            (4) Physical
                  Eating Disorders
                  Stereotyped Movement Disorders
                  Other Disorders with Physical Manifestations

            (5) Developmental
                  Pervasive Developmental Disorders
                  Specific Developmental Disorders

Each of these categories and the specific disorders they contain will be examined in depth.

INTELLECTUAL
The one major disorder in this category, Mental Retardation, focuses on impairment of intellectual functioning.

38 **Mental Retardation**
In making a diagnosis of Mental Retardation, the clinician must determine the presence of significantly subaverage general intellectual functioning which results in, or is associated with, deficits or impairments in adaptive behavior, with the onset before the age of 18.

The Mental Retardation diagnosis should be made regardless of coexisting mental or physical disorders. Other mental disorders present should also be coded on Axis I. In making a judgment of the presence of another disorder, the clinician must first subtract all the symptomatology that could be accounted for by the Mental Retardation. If the individual's symptoms are not accounted for by the Mental Retardation, another Axis I diagnosis should be used.

Intellectual functioning is considered to be significantly subaverage when the individual has an I.Q. of 70 or below on an individually administered I.Q. test. Since I.Q. measures are considered to have an error of measurement of approximately five points, any I.Q. score should be evaluated with some flexibility.

The diagnosis of Mental Retardation is not made solely on the basis of the I.Q. score. Adaptive functioning must also be impaired. Adaptive behavior refers to the relative age and cultural norms for autonomy and social responsibility.

When a known biological factor is present, it should be noted on Axis III.

When a person becomes functionally retarded before the age of 18 but it is known that she/he has had normal intelligence at one time, Dementia and Mental Retardation should both be diagnosed. Clinical Mental Retardation, developing after the age of 18, is classified as Dementia and coded under Organic Mental Disorders.

There are five subtypes of Mental Retardation:

39   **Mild Mental Retardation** indicates an I.Q. level in the 50–70 range. Approximately 80% of retarded individuals fall into this class. The term "educable" has been used to describe this group.

Moderate Retardation is applied when the I.Q. level is in the 35–49 range. Individuals classified as Moderately Retarded are considered "trainable." Approximately 12% of the retarded population is included in this group.

Severe Mental Retardation is considered when the I.Q. is in the 20–34 point range. These individuals demonstrate minimal speech and motor development and represent approximately 7% of the retarded population.

Profound Retardation applies to individuals with an I.Q. below 20. Profoundly Retarded persons require constant supervision and about 1% of the retarded fall into this subtype.

Unspecified is used if an individual is untestable and there exists a strong presumption of mental retardation.

The **Borderline Mental Retardation** of DSM-II is now classified as Borderline Intellectual Functioning under a V Code.

Other behavioral symptoms that require attention or treatment, and which do not represent another disorder (e.g., anxiety symptoms), may be recorded in the fifth digit of the diagnostic code, using the number "1." A code of "0" is used when there are no other behavioral symptoms.

BEHAVIORAL
There are two major types of behavioral disorders, Attention Deficit Disorder and Conduct Disorder.

Attention Deficit Disorder
40 This disorder is distinguished by developmentally inappropriate inattention and impulsivity. The impulsive shifting of attention is increasingly being recognized as the central deficit in children who previously were classified in terms of their hyperactive behavior.

Children with this disorder typically have attentional deficits which persist into adolescence even though excessive motor activity may subside. The term Attention Deficit Disorder is now used to encompass such terms as Hyperkinetic Reaction of Childhood, Hyperkinetic Syndrome, Hyperactive Child Syndrome, Minimal Brain Damage, Minimal Brain Dysfunction, Minimal Cerebral Dysfunction, and Minor Cerebral Dysfunction.

In cases of Mild or Moderate Mental Retardation with Attention Deficit Disorder, both diagnoses can be made on Axis I; this is not necessary with Severe or Profound Retardation.

Schizophrenia or Affective Disorder associated with symptoms of Attention Deficit Disorder preempt the diagnosis of the latter.

Children with an Attention Deficit Disorder quite commonly have certain other disorders (e.g., Conduct Disorder which is also coded on Axis I, or a Reading or Arithmetic Developmental Disorder which is coded on Axis II).

Subclasses of the Attention Deficit Disorder focus on and are coded according to the presence or absence of hyperactivity or the presence of residual effects.

Conduct Disorder
41 This disorder is characterized by a repetitive and persistent pattern of conduct which violates the basic rights of others or age appropriate societal norms or rules. To be diagnosed, the behavior must be more serious and intense than the ordinary mischief of children and adolescents.

Subclassification of the Conduct Disorder is based on the nature of the acts and on the degree of social bonding demonstrated by the individual.

Undersocialized should be considered if the child shows little or no affection, empathy, loyalties, or social bonding with others.

Socialized types demonstrate some evidence of social attachment to others.

Aggressive-nonaggressive takes into consideration whether the pattern of conduct is primarily made up of aggressive behavior, like mugging, or is primarily of a nonviolent type, such as lying or stealing.

Atypical subclass applies when the behavior violates rights or is socially age-inappropriate but it cannot be classified in one of the other subgroups.

Isolated acts of antisocial behavior (not repetitive or persistent) that have *not* impaired social and school performance should be classified under the V Code as Childhood or Adolescent Antisocial Behavior.

EMOTIONAL
There are two major classes of emotional disorders: Anxiety Disorders of Childhood or Adolescence and Other Disorders of Infancy, Childhood, or Adolescence.

42 **Anxiety Disorders of Childhood or Adolescence**
Anxiety Disorders of Childhood or Adolescence include three subclasses: Separation Anxiety, Avoidant Disorder, and Overanxious Disorder. The main characteristic of these groups is excessive anxiety manifested by fear of separation, social avoidance, or persistent and excessive worry. This category should not be used when the behavior is part of another major disorder, like Obsessive-Compulsive Disorder, Major Depression, Schizophrenia, or Pervasive Developmental Disorder.

Separation Anxiety Disorder or Avoidant Disorder should be considered if the anxiety is focused on specific situations, such as separation from significant others or avoidance of contact with strangers.

Overanxious Disorder should be used when the anxiety is demonstrated over a variety of situations.

Other Disorders of Infancy, Childhood, or Adolescence

43 This is a mixed group of disorders which were not contained in DSM-II.

Subclasses in this category are Reactive Attachment Disorder of Infancy; Schizoid Disorder of Childhood or Adolescence; Elective Mutism; Oppositional Disorder; and Identity Disorder.

Reactive Attachment Disorder of Infancy is diagnosed when clinical signs include poor emotional and physical development due to lack of adequate caretaking, with the onset before the age of eight months. Major Depression should be considered if the clinical picture develops after eight months.

Schizoid Disorder of Childhood or Adolescence applies when there is a defect in the capacity to develop social relationships that is not due to any other mental disorder, such as Conduct Disorder or a Psychotic Disorder. In contrast, children with Avoidant Disorder of Childhood or Adolescence are interested in social participation but are inhibited by anxiety, and peer interaction, once established, is enjoyed.

Elective Mutism is diagnosed when a child refuses to speak in almost all social situations, including school, despite verbal comprehension and the ability to talk.

Oppositional Disorder should be considered when there is disobedience, negativism, and provocative opposition to authority figures. Oppositionalism in an 18–36-month-old child is normal and this diagnosis should be used only if oppositional behavior persists beyond this period.

Identity Disorder is often seen during college years. It is characterized by severe personal distress regarding one's inability to reconcile aspects of the self into a relatively coherent and acceptable sense of self. There is uncertainty about such issues as long-term goals, career choice, friendship, and sexual orientation.

PHYSICAL

A fourth major grouping of Disorders Usually First Evident in Infancy, Childhood, or Adolescence focuses on impairments in physical functioning.

There are three major classifications included in this group of physical conditions: Eating Disorders, Stereotyped Movement Disorders, and Other Disorders with Physical Manifestations.

44 **Eating Disorders**
There are five subclasses of Eating Disorders.

Anorexia Nervosa involves an intense fear of becoming obese. It includes a disturbed body image with significant weight loss, resistance to maintaining normal weight and, in females, amenorrhea.

Bulimia is recurrent binge eating.

Pica is continued eating of nonnutritive substances.

Rumination Disorder of Infancy consists of repeated regurgitation without nausea or gastrointestinal illness.

Atypical Eating Disorder is a residual category.

Anorexia Nervosa and Rumination Disorder of Infancy may have an unremitting course that progresses to death.
Simple obesity which is not due to a physical disorder can be coded in the DSM-III category of Psychological Factors Affecting Physical Condition.

Stereotyped Movement Disorders
These disorders are characterized by abnormal gross motor movement and involve tics. There are five subclasses:

45 **Transient Tic Disorder** consists of recurrent, involuntary, rapid motor movements or tics which vary in intensity over weeks or months and last less than one year.

Chronic Motor Tic Disorder also consists of recurrent, involuntary, rapid motor movements or tics. They do not vary in intensity over weeks or months and last for more than one year.

Tourette's Disorder begins between the ages of two and 15 and includes the presence of recurrent multiple motor and vocal tics.

Atypical Tic Disorder is used for tics not classifiable in the previous categories. It is unknown whether this disorder and the Transient and Chronic Tic Disorders represent distinct conditions or a continuum of severity.

Atypical Stereotypical Movement Disorder is used for conditions such as rocking, repetitive hand movements, and head banging.

Other Disorders with Physical Manifestations
These disorders include categories in which the predominant disturbance is a physical dysfunction.

There is no assumption that the physical dysfunction is associated with a mental disorder or psychological conflict. Tradition dictated the inclusion of these categories.

There are five categories in this group of disorders.

46   **Stuttering** is a disruption in the rhythmic flow of speech marked by repetitions of sounds or words or by unusual hesitations in the pattern of speech.

Functional Enuresis is repeated, involuntary urination at an age when control would be expected.

Functional Encopresis involves repeated voluntary or involuntary passage of feces in inappropriate places.

Sleepwalking Disorder is marked by repeated episodes of arising from bed during sleep and walking about.

Sleep Terror Disorder involves repeated episodes of abrupt awakening from sleep with a panicky scream.

DEVELOPMENTAL
In the category of Developmental Disorders there are two subclasses: Pervasive Developmental Disorders and Specific Developmental Disorders.

Pervasive Developmental Disorders
Pervasive Developmental Disorders are characterized by distortions in the development of multiple basic psychological functions that are involved in the development of social skills and language such as attention, perception, reality-testing, and motor movement.

In the past, children with these disorders have been described by many terms: Atypical Children, Symbiotic Psychotic Children, Childhood Schizophrenia, and Autistic Children. Although these disorders may have some psychotic features, they apparently have little in common with Schizophrenia and other Psychotic Disorders of adulthood and the term "psychosis" has been avoided in DSM-III.

In Schizophrenia occurring in childhood, there will be oddities of behavior similar to those found in the Pervasive Developmental Disorders. However, to make a diagnosis of Schizophrenia, hallucinations, delusions, and loosening of associations or incoherence would need to be present.

Pervasive Developmental Disorders include three subclasses:

47 **Infantile Autism** begins *prior* to 30 months of age and is marked by a pervasive unresponsiveness to others, gross impairment in language development, and bizarre responses to aspects of the environment. Determination of the age of onset is critical to the distinction between Infantile Autism and Childhood Onset Pervasive Developmental Disorder.

Childhood Onset Pervasive Developmental Disorder involves profound disturbance in social relations and multiple oddities of behavior, all developing *after* 30 months of age and before 12 years.

Atypical Pervasive Developmental Disorder is used when there are disruptions in multiple basic psychological functions that cannot be classified as either Infantile Autism or Childhood Onset Pervasive Developmental Disorder.

The fifth digit should be used for all of the above disorders to indicate the presence of the full syndrome (code = 0) or only residual symptoms, such as inappropriate affect, social withdrawal, etc. (code = 1).

Specific Developmental Disorders (Axis II)

48 Another group of Developmental Disorders is the subclass of Specific Developmental Disorders. Although these are included in the general class of Disorders Usually First Evident in Infancy, Childhood, or Adolescence, they are actually treated as a whole separate category.

Specific Developmental Disorders are *always* coded on Axis II and include disorders of specific areas of development that are not due to another disorder. Categories include Reading, Arithmetic and Articulation Disorders, and both Mixed and Atypical Specific Disorders.

The Specific Developmental Disorders are discussed in greater depth in Chapter 22.

CASE VIGNETTE

A five-year-old boy was brought to the child guidance center. After a considerable period of denial, his parents realized that he was not developing normally. Since age three, despite normal language development, he seemed to

become distant from and uncommunicative with them. He was easily fright-
ened, at times got angry for unexplained reasons, and at other times was observed totally engrossed in stereotyped rocking behavior in his room.

Discussion Guide
The Decision Tree for Differential Diagnosis of Psychotic Features, DSM-III,
pp. 340–341, may be helpful in reviewing this case.
    The bizarre behavior and overreaction to environmental situations, lack
of affective responsivity, and the widespread impairment in functioning are
indicative of a Pervasive Developmental Disorder. Since the age of onset is
after 30 months and before 12 years of age, the Childhood Onset subclass is
most appropriate.

49   **Answer**—See Answers, Chapter 9, a.

CASE VIGNETTE
The school counselor was asked to see this 13-year-old boy for persistent tru-
ancy and smoking on school property. He was a rather popular fellow and
many peers thought of him as a "real friend." The counselor contacted his
parents and found that at home, too, there were difficulties, in that he was
frequently caught in lies and stealing money from his mother's purse.

Discussion Guide
The Decision Tree for Differential Diagnosis of Antisocial, Aggressive, Defiant, or Oppositional Behavior, DSM-III, p. 345, may be helpful in reviewing
this case.
    The predominant problem of this child lies in the area of his behavior
where he shows a pattern that violates the rights of others, thus a Conduct
Disorder. His ability to make friends and form social bonds supports the Socialized subtype. The fact that his behavior was not of a violent, aggressive
nature indicates the Nonaggressive subtype of Conduct Disorder.

50   **Answer**—See Answers, Chapter 9, b.

Chapter 10

Substance Use Disorders and Organic Mental Disorders

GENERAL OVERVIEW

Classification systems traditionally separate disorders associated with tangible factors such as brain diseases, toxic conditions, and drug addiction.

Substance Use Disorders and Organic Mental Disorders are discussed together here because they are often clinically interrelated.

In the clinical situation, the diagnostician may be confronted with a recognizable organic syndrome which stems from disturbed brain tissue function. That disturbance could be the consequence of substance use or abuse, primary diseases in the brain, or effects of systemic physical diseases. Attention to the causative process might require definitive treatment of the physical disease or might involve correcting a harmful pattern of drug or alcohol ingestion.

DSM-III requires that there be a diagnosis for problems of abnormal substance consumption *as well as* a diagnosis of any brain syndrome that might exist as the consequence of the ingestion.

SUBSTANCE USE DISORDERS

With this class of disorders, the clinician is applying a diagnostic label to an unhealthy pattern of drug, chemical, or alcohol consumption. This is a diagnosis of the substance-consuming behavior.

Since alcohol and drugs can be consumed in a healthy manner with no problems, it is important to first define when "use" of a substance has become "abnormal use" or a use disorder. Use of a chemical, alcohol, or drug is considered normal if the agent is prescribed for legitimate medical purposes, or if it is consumed for recreational purposes without any complications of the use. The legal status of the substance has nothing to do with this distinction. Arrest for possession or consumption of an agent does not constitute a mental disorder. One may recall the distinction between mental disorder and social deviance.

52   **Substance Abuse** is a milder version of Substance Use Disorder and has to be distinguished from simple use.

A single bad encounter with the agent does not constitute a disorder. A pattern of pathological use must be defined for at least a month and there has to be an impairment in social or occupational functioning as a result. This pattern has to be verified against what is typical and normal for this person's subcultural context and found to be beyond acceptable limits. The person may be staying under the influence all day long or may indulge in uncontrolled binges.

Substance Dependence is when the abnormal consumption becomes more serious than Abuse. This distinction requires that the criteria for Abuse have already been met and that there is evidence of tolerance and/or withdrawal.

Tolerance is indicated when the person must considerably increase the dose to maintain the same degree of effect.

Withdrawal symptoms are evident when, with cessation or reduction of intake, there is a rebound process that includes physiological upset as well as profound craving for the withdrawn substance.

With either Abuse or Dependence, the clinician must designate in the fifth digit one of the following patterns of intake:

53   **Continuous:**   1—regular use for over six months
       Episodic: 2—a pattern of short periods (binges)
       In Remission: 3—not now taking substance in maladaptive fashion
       Unspecified: 0—course unknown or yet uncertain

In classifying the Substance Use Disorder, the type of substance is the basis for the designation. (There is an official listing of substance types, with separate codes for Abuse and Dependence. See DSM-III, p. 17.) As noted in Table 6, some types of substances, such as alcohol, can produce dependence, while others, such as cocaine, do not.

The classification appears formidable; however, the use of the system is simple:

- First, name the actual substance involved.
- Then, note the degree of use (Abuse or Dependence).
- This is followed by the pattern of intake to complete the diagnosis.
- For example, LSD Abuse, Episodic.

For those involved in coding the records, it is important to realize that the class *Amphetamine or Similarly Acting Sympathomimetic* includes diet pills and stimulants like Ritalin. One writes only the name of the substance (i.e., Ritalin Abuse, not the tongue twister name of the class).

TABLE 6
Substance Abuse and Dependence

Alcohol	abuse _____	305.0X
	dependence _____	303.9X
"Barbiturate or Similarly Acting	abuse _____	305.4X
Sedative or Hypnotic"	dependence _____	304.1X
Opioid	abuse _____	305.5X
	dependence _____	304.0X
Cocaine	abuse _____	305.6X
"Amphetamine or Similarly Acting	abuse _____	305.7X
Sympathomimetic"	dependence _____	304.4X
Phencyclidine (PCP) or Similarly	abuse _____	305.9X
Acting Arylcyclohexylamine		
Hallucinogen	abuse _____	305.3X
Cannabis	abuse _____	305.2X
	dependence _____	304.3X
Tobacco	dependence _____	305.1X
Other	abuse _____	305.9X
	dependence _____	304.6X

Barbiturate or Similarly Acting Sedative or Hypnotic includes not only outright sedatives but also mild tranquilizers like Valium.

Glue sniffing would be coded as *Other Specified Substance.*

An example of the way a complete Substance Use Disorder diagnosis is recorded on Axis I is: Dalmane Dependence, Continuous (304.11).

CASE VIGNETTE

A 25-year-old housewife with insomnia obtained a prescription for 10 mg Valium from her family physician, who also prescribed the medication for the patient's mother. The patient found that two pills at bedtime brought satisfying sleep, but she raised the dose to three just to be sure she had enough. Then, she started taking the medicine during the day for relaxation. For about three months, two pills during the day were sufficient, but for the last four months the drug seemed to lose its effectiveness. Consequently, she was taking four and then five pills through the daytime. She had to consume her mother's supply as well as her own, and to pretend that she'd lost a prescription or two in order to secure a sufficient supply. The mother raised objections, but the patient declared that she couldn't cope without the Valium, and that she only craved it more when she tried to cut down. Despite her claim of coping, the patient's husband declared that she was "zonked out" all day and didn't keep up with the housework.

Discussion Guide

This answer can be discussed by citing the use of Valium in the diagnosis, the evidence of tolerance and withdrawal, and the continuous pattern of ingestion.

54   **Answer**—See Answers, Chapter 10, a.

ORGANIC MENTAL DISORDERS

55   Several disorders illustrate an overlap of psychiatry with neurology. Drug abuse, the residual effect of a drug, cessation of a tolerated drug, a toxic agent, primary brain degeneration, a circulatory disorder, systemic disease and/or neurologic disease can all affect the brain.

56   The brain is an organ which produces mental activity. Derangement in that organ will result in it producing disordered mental activity, called Organic Brain Syndromes.

There are nine identified syndromes which can be clinically distinguished based on the extent, nature, and duration of underlying brain pathology. Sometimes, one syndrome may follow or be superimposed on another.

The diagnostician must first recognize and properly label the syndrome. The classification is then made according to the etiologic process. The syndromes are arranged in a hierarchy, with the simplest syndromes at the top and the more complex at the bottom.

If the features of a more complex syndrome are present, that diagnosis generally takes precedence over the simpler syndrome. The first two syndromes, Intoxication and Withdrawal, can only be drug-induced; the remaining seven can have either origin.

Table 7 lists the nine syndromes and indicates their possible cause(s).

Intoxication

This syndrome involves the recent ingestion and presence in the body of something that produces the intoxication symptoms. The precise features will depend on the substance ingested, whether it is a stimulant or a depressant, an upper or a downer.

Social drinking that would be called "intoxication" by a physiologist would not qualify as a mental disorder. For the diagnosis of a mental disorder to be considered, there must be a maladaptive effect, such as developing problems in work or social relationships.

TABLE 7
Drug- and/or Disease-Induced Syndromes

Drug-Induced	Syndromes	Disease-Induced
x	Intoxication	
x	Withdrawal	
x	Organic Personality Syndrome	x
x	Organic Affective Syndrome	x
x	Organic Hallucinosis	x
x	Organic Delusional Syndrome	x
x	Organic Amnestic Syndrome	x
x	Dementia	x
x	Delirium	x

If a person's intoxication process goes further, to the production of more complex symptoms, the more complex diagnosis takes precedence.

Withdrawal

The Withdrawal Syndrome occurs when an individual with a Substance Dependence Disorder curtails intake of the tolerated drug, resulting in a rebound phenomenon with physiological symptoms and a profound desire for the curtailed substance. The nature of the rebound depends on the drug on which the individual was dependent.

The label of Withdrawal applies if the clinical picture includes only the features of the rebound phenomenon. If the rebound process generates more complex symptoms, the more complex diagnosis prevails.

Organic Personality Syndrome

The Organic Personality Syndrome involves a marked change in personality, with a dulling, coarsening or social deterioration. The individual may show exaggeration of previous undesirable traits, as well as socially inappropriate actions, without regard for the consequences.

This syndrome should be considered whenever one sees a drastic change in a person who has a lifelong history of stable character patterns. These individuals often show emotional lability, impaired impulse control, apathy, or indifference. Occasionally they are defensive and suspicious.

Sometimes this syndrome is the first evidence of brain degeneration. When intellectual deterioration shows up, the diagnosis should be changed to one of Dementia.

Organic Affective Syndrome

In this syndrome, mood is deranged on an organic basis. The mood derangement constitutes a manic or a depressive syndrome. The severity of the mood disorder may range from mild to psychotic.

The usual cause is toxic or metabolic. Certain antihypertensive drugs are notorious for inducing a depression (i.e., Reserpine and Aldomet). Hormonal disorders are another cause (i.e., adrenal or thyroid glands), along with viral illness such as mononucleosis and influenza.

If symptoms any more complex than mood disturbance appear, a more complex diagnosis is required.

Organic Hallucinosis

This syndrome features hallucinations that occur in a fully awake and alert state. The hallucinations are generally auditory or visual, depending somewhat on the organic process involved. The experience of hallucinations in clear consciousness may be pleasant or terrifying. The hallucinations may be identified by the individual as real or unreal.

The most common causes of this syndrome are hallucinogen abuse, sensory deprivation, and alcohol abuse (nutritional).

The person may believe that the hallucinations are real, but any more elaborate delusions would require the more complex diagnosis of Organic Delusional Syndrome.

Any impairment of sensorium would require a diagnosis of Delirium.

Organic Delusional Syndrome

Organic Delusional Syndrome occurs if there are organic reasons for delusions taking place in a state of clear consciousness. The delusions may be chaotic or highly organized. This delusional syndrome can be produced by amphetamines, hallucinogens, marijuana, seizure disorder, and degenerative brain diseases.

These states may be clinically indistinguishable from paranoid delusional states of a purely functional origin. If a paranoid delusional state appears in a person over 30 who has never shown a mental problem before, both an Organic Delusional Syndrome and Paranoia should be considered.

Organic Amnestic Syndrome

This syndrome emphasizes memory impairment without the complexity of Dementia or Delirium.

The individual can retain information only as long as he can sustain attention on it. He will be able to recall an event right after it occurs but not after the subject has changed for a few minutes. There will be some disorientation, but awareness of self and surroundings is intact.

These individuals are apt to be bland and apathetic. Sometimes they are friendly but shallow. They almost always minimize, conceal, or deny the defect in memory.

The usual cause is nutritional, such as a vitamin deficiency in drinkers/ alcoholics.

Dementia

This syndrome contains the features of the Amnestic Syndrome, but includes more extensive symptoms which result in deterioration from previous levels of function and intelligence. The decline must be sufficient to impair social or occupational functioning. In addition to memory impairment, there is impaired abstraction and judgment, cognitive defects, and personality change.

The course is a stable downhill progression, and sensorium is not disturbed. This helps to distinguish Dementia from Delirium.

Although there may be other causes, most cases of Dementia are caused by brain degeneration from neurological diseases such as Alzheimer's, Pick's, or cerebrovascular disease.

Delirium

Unlike Dementia, this is a rapidly develping, considerably fluctuating, complex syndrome in which sensorium is *not clear.*

Attention, memory, orientation, perception, level of wakefulness, and psychomotor activity are all affected. The most prominent feature is impaired attention; sometimes it can be focused for only a moment. The person switches from subject to subject losing the train of thought. Thinking will be slowed or accelerated. Reasoning and goal-directed behavior are impossible. Memory and orientation are impaired, and they may be untestable because the person can't sustain attention.

Awareness of surroundings is lost so that strange places and faces may be taken to be familiar. There is a fluctuating sensorium, with drowsiness or excessive wakefulness. Vivid dreams, nightmares, misperceptions, illusions, and hallucinations are common. There is a variable subjective state ranging from terror to apathy to rage. The disorder is generally worse at night, in the dark, or when alone.

There may be lucid intervals as the patient moves towards recovery. The course is a quick recovery or a quick decline to coma and death. There is a multiplicity of causes, especially toxic and metabolic.

CLASSIFICATION

The syndromes just reviewed are not in themselves diagnoses. The diagnostic process involves recognition and proper labeling of the syndrome, then linking that to the causal process.

Subclassification of Organic Mental Disorders takes into account the causal process by setting up three groupings:

57

(1) Senile and Presenile Dementia

(2) Substance-induced syndromes

(3) Cause is a disease which is unknown, or is some physical disease other than those involved in Senile and Presenile Dementias. The causative disease process will be listed on Axis III.

Senile and Presenile Dementias

58 The first subgrouping puts together the Senile and Presenile Dementias (these are not the only Dementia Syndromes).

Primary Degenerative Dementia stems from direct decay of brain tissue.

Multi-infarct Dementia stems from cerebrovascular disease which produces a series of little strokes with patchy destruction of brain tissue.

For a complete diagnosis, the Senile and Presenile Dementias must be labeled according to presence or absence of associated features (delirium, delusions, depression, or uncomplicated) which involves syndromes superimposed on the Dementia.

Substance-induced Mental Disorders

The second grouping is Substance-induced Organic Mental Disorders. The substance types are almost exactly the same as for Substance Use Disorders.

As Table 8 indicates, some substances can induce a variety of syndromes, others only one or two.

TABLE 8
Substance-induced Syndromes

Substance	Syndromes
Alcohol	7
"Barbiturate or Similarly Acting Sedative"	4
Opioid	2
Cocaine	Intoxication Only
"Amphetamine or Similarly Acting Sympathomimetic"	4
Phencyclidine (PCP) or Similarly Acting Arylcyclohexylamine	3
Hallucinogen	3
Cannabis	2
Tobacco	Withdrawal Only
Caffeine	Intoxication Only
Other or Unspecified Substance	10

Again, one names the actual substance, not the tongue twisting official name of the class of drug.

Syndromes Caused by Known or Unknown Physical Conditions
The third grouping is for syndromes caused by a disease or physical condition other than those in Senile and Presenile Dementia. The physical condition, including neurological disorders, is named on Axis III.

59   These include: Delirium, Dementia, Amnestic Syndrome, Organic Delusional Syndrome, Organic Hallucinosis, Organic Affective Syndrome, Organic Personality Syndrome, and Atypical or Mixed Organic Brain Syndrome. This grouping is also used when the organic syndrome is caused by a condition which cannot be identified.

CASE VIGNETTE
A 43-year-old, divorced, housepainter is examined in the hospital emergency observation ward. His sister is available to provide some information. The sister indicates that the patient has consumed large quantities of cheap wine, daily, for five years. Evidently, he had a reasonably stable home life and job record until his wife left him for another man five years ago. The sister indicates that the patient drinks more than a fifth a day, and that this has been a pattern since the divorce. He has often had blackouts from drinking, missed work, and consequently has been fired from several jobs. Fortunately, painters are in great demand and he has been able to provide marginally for himself during these years. However, three days ago he ran out of money and has had to beg on the street to buy a meal. He has been very poorly nourished, eating perhaps one meal a day and evidently relying on the wine as his primary source of nourishment.

The morning after his last day of drinking he felt increasingly tremulous, with his hands shaking so grossly that it was difficult for him to light a cigarette. Accompanying this was an increasing sense of inner panic which has made him virtually unable to sleep. A neighbor became concerned about the patient when he seemed not to be making sense and was clearly unable to take care of himself. The neighbor contacted the sister who brought the patient to the hospital.

On examination, he alternates between apprehension and chatty superficial warmth. He is quite keyed up and talks constantly. At times he recognizes the doctor, but sometimes he thinks that the doctor is the patient's older brother. Twice during the examination the patient called the doctor by his older brother's name and asked when he had arrived, evidently having lost track of the interview up to that point. There is a gross hand tremor at rest and there are periods of picking at bugs he sees on the bedsheets. The patient is disoriented regarding time and thinks that he is in a supermarket parking lot rather than in a hospital. He indicates that he feels he is fighting against a terrifying sense that the world is ending in a holocaust. He is startled every few minutes by sounds and scenes of fiery car crashes (based on the sound of rolling carts in the hall). Efforts at testing memory and calculation fail because his attention shifts too quickly to sustain the effort. An electroencephalogram indicates a pattern of diffuse encephalopathy.

Discussion Guide
The use of the Decision Tree for Differential Diagnosis of Organic Brain Syndromes, DSM-III, p. 349, can facilitate this review.

In diagnosing this case it is important to recognize the features of delirium, noting that alcohol withdrawal is the substance-induced process involved. This is the new official term for the old "delirium tremens."

60 **Answer**—See Answers, Chapter 10, b.

ignor Chapter 11

Schizophrenic Disorders, Psychotic Disorders Not Elsewhere Classified, and Paranoid Disorders

GENERAL CONCEPTS ABOUT THESE CLASSES

These three classes border on each other in the classification sequence and in the actual clinical situation.

DSM-III uses the term "psychotic" to mean a condition which includes a loss of contact with reality. Psychotic conditions may be found in Organic Mental Disorders (Delirium, for example); Disorders Usually First Evident in Infancy, Childhood, or Adolescence (Pervasive Developmental Disorder, for example); extreme cases of Affective Disorders (Mania, for example); and in this set of classes, which apply to the bulk of psychotic conditions encountered.

All of the disorders in these classes involve, at some point in the illness, the prominent presence of hallucinations, delusions, severely deranged behavior, or markedly disrupted thinking.

SCHIZOPHRENIC DISORDERS

Essential Features

Until now, Schizophrenia was defined inconsistently in this country; one clinician would use the term only for a disabling florid psychosis, while another

70

would apply the term to nonpsychotic individuals with hazy and subtle peculiarities in their self-experience and thinking.

Diagnostic criteria used in research over the past decade have assisted in defining these conditions in a manner that provides for more general agreement and understanding.

Schizophrenic Disorders in DSM-III are serious illnesses. There is a tendency for: familial transmission; onset in early adulthood; a precipitate drop from an established level of functioning; a characteristic set of symptoms that involve aberration in a whole array of mental functions; recurrences and further disability; and a characteristic response to reasonably specific treatment approaches.

A person with Schizophrenia will have had, at some point in time, capacity to function on a par with "normal" people. With the onset of the illness, there is either a plummeting drop or a deteriorating downward slide to a level similar to that of a retarded or demented person.

If this kind of clinical picture is due to a definable organic process, then a diagnosis of Organic Mental Disorder would take precedence.

Sometimes a severe Affective Disorder can so disrupt a person's mental and personal functioning that a picture transiently on a par with Schizophrenia is produced. When the clinical picture seems to be accounted for by an Affective Disorder, the diagnosis of Affective Disorder takes precedence over a diagnosis of Schizophrenia. This distinction requires not only that the mood is prominently disturbed, but that the mood disturbance is the primary and original derangement, with other features following along later.

Characteristic Symptoms

61 Schizophrenia produces widespread havoc in the personality and a whole range of functions will be affected. No single symptom establishes the diagnosis. The coexistence of disturbances in the following areas can be a clue to the diagnostician that this may be Schizophrenia.

Communication. It is generally from communication that inferences about a person's thinking can be drawn. Usually the first thing that strikes the clinician is that these people don't make sense when they talk. Both spoken and written communication are deranged, with language that doesn't follow the rules, and with talk that presents obstacles to a listener's immediate understanding.

Commonly, things may be said in juxtaposition, but lacking any comprehensible relationship. Talk may be vague, repetitive, or stereotyped, and facts may be put together with faultily drawn conclusions. The thought proc-

esses may be so disorganized that speech is a stream of incoherent words.
It has to be established that this person made sense before the onset of the disorder to, for example, make the distinction from Mental Retardation.

Thought Content. Things are going on in a schizophrenic's head that are not going on in other people's. A set of highly characteristic delusions may be present, and can be a tip-off to the diagnosis. Bizarre delusions that are physically or utterly implausible, such as delusions of being controlled by external forces or delusions that one's thoughts are being broadcast, are strongly suggestive of Schizophrenia and aid in ruling out other disorders.

Perception. Schizophrenics may hear, see, feel, smell, and taste things that are not there. The most common perceptual derangement in Schizophrenia is auditory hallucinations, but a whole variety of illusions, including illusory somatic experience, as well as various hallucinations, may be present.

Affect. The normal "showing-through" of emotions may be affected so that the person generates an uncanny or eerie impact on the observer. Display of emotions or affect may be blunted, inappropriate, or unpredictably variable.

Self-experience. These people may have lost touch with who they are. There may be doubts, concerns, and worries over "just who am I?" The comfortable sense of certainty about oneself may no longer be taken for granted. The person may feel that the very core of his identity is vulnerable or changing in some mysterious way. For example, a man may feel he's being changed into a woman.

Motivation—Vitality—Drive. Energy, enthusiasm, and effort may be abnormally increased, sometimes to a level of sheer excitement. On the other hand, a person's drive and sense of direction may be lost or squelched.

Social Engagement. The person may withdraw, like a hermit, from other people. The person may be so withdrawn from the world that he/she is absorbed entirely in his/her mixed-up thoughts.

Motor Behavior. The person may be visibly abnormal from across the room. There may be odd appearance, pacing, running amok, statue-like rigid posturing, or bizarre mannerisms.

Subjective Comfort. A variety of subjective distress may be present as one of the most prominent features. There may be anguish, frantic desperation or abysmal despair. Less dramatically, there may be unrest, apathy, or ennui.

Onset and Course

There are usually some events in the person's life that trigger the development or exacerbation of the disorder. When precipitating influences are known, those psychosocial stressors should be identified and rated on Axis IV.

The onset may be abrupt, with sudden florid psychosis. More typically, there is a prodromal period with fairly low-grade but distinct symptoms. Following the prodromal period, there is a stage of florid psychosis with prominent hallucinations, delusions, or deranged thought processes. When the stage of florid psychosis settles, there is often a stage of residual symptoms rather like the prodromal period. The patient may lose the fresh turmoil of the active psychotic phase and become "burned-out," lifeless.

Schizophrenia is being defined as a subchronic or chronic disorder. The period of continuous illness, including prodrome, active, and residual phases, must persist for more than six months.

The person may not make a full recovery to normality and his/her previous high level of functioning. He/she may be vulnerable to recurrences of the full-blown disorder. When there are recurrences, there is usually some loss in the level of functioning after each florid episode. Thus the long range course is, stepwise, downward.

The person may recover and overcome all symptoms of illness in that he/she can be declared "in remission," meaning that there are no residual symptoms. If, after a long period of remission, the patient is not fragile and vulnerable to recurrences and can sustain that state without treatment, the diagnosis may be changed from Schizophrenia, In Remission, to No Disorder. That decision requires a high level of clinical judgment.

To meet the criteria, people with acute psychotic episodes can no longer be diagnosed Schizophrenic. Those whose illnesses last less than six months, even repeatedly, are to be classified under Psychotic Disorders Not Elsewhere Classified.

Persons who never develop the full-blown psychotic state cannot be called Schizophrenic. There is no longer a nonpsychotic type of Schizophrenia for those cases which in the past would have been called Latent Schizophrenia, Simple Schizophrenia, and Pseudoneurotic Schizophrenia. One must now consider a diagnosis of Personality Disorder for such cases.

A boundary has been defined so that the diagnosis of Schizophrenic Disorder is used only if the onset is before age 45. An identical condition with onset after that age would be called Atypical Psychosis.

Diagnostic Criteria
There are six criteria for the diagnosis of Schizophrenia identified as A through F in DSM-III, pp. 188–190, and in Table 9.

- Criterion A concentrates on the cross-sectional exam of mental status. It only takes one of these items to meet criterion A. These are used

TABLE 9
Diagnostic Criteria for Schizophrenia

A. At least one of the following at some point in the illness:

(1) Bizarre delusions
(2) Somatic, grandiose, religious, nihilistic or other delusions (not persecutory or jealous)
(3) Persecutory or jealous delusions if accompanied by hallucinations of any type
(4) Auditory hallucinations
(5) Incoherence, markedly illogical thoughts, or marked poverty of content in speech if associated with one:
a. blunted, flat, or inappropriate affect
b. delusions or hallucinations
c. catatonic or other grossly deranged behavior

B. Deterioration in adaptive functioning

C. Symptoms are present and have been continuous for more than six months

D. Affective Disorder ruled out

E. Onset before age 45

F. Organicity and Mental Retardation ruled out

as an important set of distinctions in differential diagnosis to distinguish Schizophrenia from an actual Paranoid Disorder.

• Criterion B requires the all-important loss of adaptive functioning.
• Criterion C relates to duration.
• Criterion D indicates that Affective Disorder must be excluded.
• Criterion E is the arbitrary age limit for onset.
• Criterion F excludes organicity. If Mental Retardation is present, as much of the clinical picture that is explainable as features of retardation would be credited to that disorder. If sufficient symptoms beyond the bounds of retardation are present, both diagnoses are made.

These criteria are the guides to the class of Schizophrenia. Schizophrenia is not in itself a complete diagnosis; a complete diagnosis requires designation of the type of Schizophrenia and the course of the condition.

Types

62 There are five types of Schizophrenia based on the differentiation of the cluster of symptoms into some distinctive pattern. Each type must first meet the criteria for the class of Schizophrenia.

Disorganized Type. Features of this type include prominent incoherence, lack of systematized delusions, and blunted, inappropriate, or silly affect. This is the type when the clinical picture has differentiated toward incoherence as the prominent feature.

Catatonic Type. Features of the Catatonic Type include stupor or mutism, negativism, rigidity, excitement, and posturing. This is the type when the clinical picture has differentiated into some of these rather dramatic features.

Paranoid Type. Features of this type are persecutory and grandiose delusions, delusional jealousy, and persecutory or grandiose hallucinations. If the clinical picture has differentiated into a great deal of paranoid organization, this is the type of Schizophrenia. First of all, there must be the features that establish that this is Schizophrenia, then that it fits this Paranoid Type. A Paranoid Disorder could not meet the criteria for Schizophrenia.

Undifferentiated Type. This type of Schizophrenia features grossly disorganized behavior, hallucinations, incoherence, or prominent delusions. This category is used when the criteria for other types are not met, or an individual meets the criteria for more than one of the other types. This type has not differentiated in a clear-cut way into any of the other types. This category is not meant to allow for evasion of a distinct diagnosis, nor should it be used as a wastebasket term.

Residual Type. This diagnosis is used when there are no prominent criterion A symptoms present when the person is seen, but these symptoms have been present at least one time in the past. At the time the person is seen, there are only residual symptoms. There may be some delusions and hallucinations, but the person is "burned-out" and there is not the fresh turmoil of the florid active phase.

Residual Type often applies to chronic outpatients who are still exhibiting some symptoms of the disorder. This should be the designated type when there are some symptoms and the clinician is tempted to say that the person is in a "partial remission." However, the term "partial remission" is not an acceptable one. It is necessary to designate that the diagnosis is now Residual Type. Individuals designated this type could have been classified as some other type earlier in the illness.

Course

63   To complete the diagnosis, the course of the illness must be indicated after the type. Designation of the course involves a combination of duration and presence or absence of symptoms.

Subchronic means continuous illness more than six months but less than two years.

Subchronic with Acute Exacerbation is the same time interval as subchronic, but the individual has been in the residual state and has become psychotic again.

Chronic means continuous illness lasting more than two years.

Chronic with Acute Exacerbation is the same time frame as chronic, but the individual had been in the residual state and has become psychotic again.

In Remission means that there are no symptoms now; the patient must be free of all symptoms, including residual ones. The person may or may not be receiving medication while designated "in remission." There is no such designation as "partial remission."

CASE VIGNETTE

A 16-year-old boy moved from a small rural school to a large urban high school for his junior year. Without voicing any lack of confidence about handling this new situation, he became increasingly less communicative over the course of that school year. His grades, which had been all B's and C's, fell to D's and D – 's. Through the following summer, his family noticed that he seemed to have changed, to have become withdrawn into himself. He tended to give laconic responses and sometimes had an inscrutable expression on his face. Two weeks after the senior year began, the boy became so disturbed in the classroom that school authorities contacted his parents, who brought him to the hospital the next week. He appears rather stunned and perplexed, and his tone of voice is flat and mechanical. Occasionally, he contorts his face into a grimace and twirls the hair of his right temple between his thumb and fingers. He moves easily about and complies with instructions. He is verbal, but his speech is like "word salad," just an incoherent jumble of words. He seems to try to listen to questions, but his answers are a stream of incoherent speech. He seems at times to be hearing voices or other sounds, in that his eyes dart to the side and he adopts a listening attitude.

Discussion Guide
This case can be reviewed using the Decision Tree for Differential Diagnosis of Psychotic Features, DSM-III, pp. 340–341.

Note that the criteria for Schizophrenia are met, that the prominent incoherence helps to designate this type as disorganized, and that the time frame and pattern, prodrome and fresh psychotic symptoms match a subchronic course.

64 **Answer**—See Answers, Chapter 11, a.

PSYCHOTIC DISORDERS NOT ELSEWHERE CLASSIFIED
65 There are four Psychotic Disorders that are not classified elsewhere. They are: Brief Reactive Psychosis, Schizophreniform Disorder, Schizoaffective Disorder, and Atypical Psychosis.

The first two have a cross-sectional picture that meets all the criteria for Schizophrenia, except for the duration. The second two, Schizoaffective and Atypical Psychosis, are special categories for differential diagnostic problems.

Each of these is already a complete diagnosis and there is no need to provide type or course.

Brief Reactive Psychosis
Brief Reactive Psychosis will occur in an individual who was doing fine until he/she encountered some overwhelming stress, which threw him/her abruptly into a psychotic state.

This condition was unofficially called "three-day schizophrenia" in the past. The picture resolves promptly, with no inclination to further problems. If the condition does persist past two weeks, the diagnosis should be changed to the next category, Schizophreniform Disorder.

Schizophreniform Disorder

Schizophreniform Disorder is the label used for acute psychotic breaks that were once labeled "acute schizophrenic episode." These are usually sharp psychotic breaks without a gradual prodrome.

There tends to be a lot of turmoil in the picture, and the prognosis is generally good. The entire illness, despite the severity of the symptoms, runs its course in less than six months. If the condition persists past six months, the diagnosis should be changed to Schizophrenia.

Schizoaffective Disorder

The category of Schizoaffective Disorder is more a statement than a diagnosis per se. Sometimes the diagnostician finds a case where, for some reason, it simply is not possible to make a clear distinction between Affective Disorder and Schizophrenia.

Atypical Psychosis

The category of Atypical Psychosis is used for:

- Psychotic Disorders that fail to meet the exact criteria for other diagnoses, such as "Schizophrenia" developing after age 45.
- a Psychotic Disorder that seems to have its own unique features, such as certain monosymptomatic psychotic states.
- a recognizable Psychotic Disorder where the clinician is not yet able to distinguish exactly which disorder is present. The diagnosis can be changed when more information clarifies the story.

CASE VIGNETTE

A 42-year-old socialite has never had any psychiatric disturbance before. A new performance hall is to be formally opened by presenting the world premiere of a ballet. The woman, because of her position on the cultural council, has taken on the responsibility for coordinating that event. However, construction problems, including strikes, have made it uncertain that the finishing details will meet the deadline. The set designer has been volatile, threatening to walk out on the project unless the materials meet his meticulous specifications. The woman has had to attempt to cool down this volatile man, while attempting to coax the negotiations between the disputing groups. She also has increased responsibilities at home in that her housekeeper has had to leave to visit a sick relative.

In the midst of this tension and turmoil, the woman's best friend is killed and almost decapitated in a tragic auto crash. The woman herself is an only child and her best friend had been very close to her since grade school. People had often commented that the two women were like sisters. Immediately following the funeral, the woman becomes increasingly tense and jittery, only able to sleep two or three hours a night. Two days later the patient happens to see a woman driving a car just like the one that her friend had. She immediately becomes puzzled, and after a few hours she becomes convinced that her friend is alive and that the accident and funeral were staged as part of a plot. Somehow the plot is directed toward deceiving her and she senses that she is in great danger and must solve the mystery to escape alive. She begins to distrust everyone except her husband, and senses that the phone is tapped and the rooms are "bugged." She pleads with her husband to help save her life. She is starting to hear a high-pitched undulating sound, which she fears may be a beam of ultrasound aimed at her. She is in a state of sheer panic, gripping her husband's arm in terror as he brings her to the emergency room the next morning.

Discussion Guide
This case can be reviewed using the Decision Tree for Differential Diagnosis of Psychotic Features, DSM-III, pp. 340–341.

Note the overwhelming stressor, the death of a friend, to be listed on Axis IV, the turmoil in work relations, the florid acute psychotic state, and the time frame.

66   **Answer**—See Answers, Chapter 11, b.

PARANOID DISORDERS
67   The Paranoid Disorders are psychotic states that are best understood in juxtaposition to the other Psychotic Disorders previously covered. What distinguishes the Paranoid Disorders is that they do not have all the symptoms to meet the criteria for other disorders. They simply feature an organized delusional system in an otherwise more or less intact individual.

These cases feature no prominent hallucinations, only persecutory delusions or delusional jealousy. The delusions in Paranoid Disorders must be plausible. They cannot be the bizarre, physically impossible delusions of

Schizophrenia and related psychoses. The duration of symptoms must be at least one week.

Emotion and behavior may be somewhat disturbed, but will be consistent with the deluded thinking (indignation, revenge, counterattacks). There is not the marked drop in functioning found in Schizophrenia, and routine daily occupational functioning is generally intact.

The onset of Paranoid Disorder tends to be somewhat later in life than Schizophrenia. Since paranoid symptoms can be a prominent part of organic conditions, those are ruled out before considering a diagnosis of Paranoid Disorder.

The four disorders within this classification, all of which must meet the criteria for Paranoid Disorder, are Paranoia, Acute Paranoid Disorder, Shared Paranoid Disorder, and Atypical Paranoid Disorder.

Paranoia
The central diagnosis in this class is called Paranoia. It features persistent persecutory delusions or delusional jealousy of at least six months' duration.

Acute Paranoid Disorder
Acute Paranoid Disorder meets the same criteria as Paranoia; however, the duration is less than six months. If the condition persists past six months, the diagnosis should be changed to Paranoia.

Shared Paranoid Disorder
This is the diagnosis for someone who has a close relationship with a person who has an established paranoid psychotic state of any class. Through this involvement, the impressionable person adopts the delusions of the paranoid person.

This state of affairs has been called "folie à deux" in the past. The diagnosis of Shared Paranoid Disorder is given only to the impressionable person of the pair. The diagnosis of the dominant person would depend on the exact nature of his/her disorder, for example, Paranoid Schizophrenia.

Atypical Paranoid Disorder
This category is for a Paranoid Disorder that does not quite fit any of the other subtypes.

CASE VIGNETTE
A beautiful, successful, 34-year-old interior designer is brought to the clinic by her 37-year-old husband, a rather prominent attorney. The husband

laments that for the past three years his wife has made increasingly shrill accusations that he is unfaithful to her. He declares that he has done everything in his power to convince her of his innocence, but there is no shaking her conviction. A careful examination of the facts reveals that there is actually no evidence that the man has been unfaithful. When asked what her evidence is, she becomes somewhat vague and mysterious, declaring that she can tell by such things as a faraway look in his eyes.

She is absolutely sure that she is right and considers herself highly insulted to be told that she is imagining the disloyalty. The husband reports that for the last year she has been increasingly bitter, creating a kind of "cold war" atmosphere in the household. Militantly entrenched against the husband and refusing to show him any affection except at social gatherings, she seems intent on giving the impression socially that they have a good relationship. However, after they are alone, the coldness reenters the picture. She has actually physically assaulted the husband on occasion, but her account obscures the fact that she initiated the assault. Her description of the tussles actually begin with the point where the husband attempted to interrupt her assault by holding her arms. She declares that she will never forgive him for holding her down and squeezing her arms, and her account makes it appear that she was unfairly pinned down by the husband.

The patient experiences no hallucinations; her speech is well organized; she interprets proverbs with no difficulty; she seems to have a good command of current events; and generally she displays no difficulty with thinking, aside from her conviction of the disloyalty. She describes herself as having a generally full and effective life, with a few close friends and no problems except those centering on her experiences of unhappiness in the marriage. The husband reports that his wife is respected for her skills but that she has had difficulties for most of her life in close relationships with friends. She has lost a number of friends because she seems always to be intolerant of differences in opinion. The woman reports that she does not want to leave the marriage, nor does she want to have her husband leave her; instead she is furious about the injustice and she demands that it be confessed and redeemed.

Discussion Guide

This case can be reviewed by utilizing the Decision Tree for Differential Diagnosis of Psychotic Features, DSM-III, pp. 340–341. Note that the criteria for other psychoses are not met, that the criteria for delusional jealousy are met, and that the time frame covers more than six months.

68 **Answer**—See Answers, Chapter 11, c.

Chapter 12

Affective Disorders

GENERAL OVERVIEW

69 All of the disorders in this classification have, as a common denominator, a primary and preponderant disturbance in *mood.* Mood is a prolonged and pervasive emotional state that affects the total person: feelings, outlook, attitude, self-regard, activity level, homeostatic balance, and trends in thinking.

The Affective Disorders classification is only concerned with excessively low or high moods. This class of disorders is divided into three subclasses: Major Affective Disorders, Other Specific Affective Disorders, and Atypical Affective Disorders.

Major Affective Disorders include Bipolar Disorder and Major Depression. They are distinguished by a full affective syndrome and whether or not there has ever been a manic episode.

Other Specific Affective Disorders are characterized by a partial affective syndrome of at least two years' duration. This class includes Cyclothymic and Dysthymic Disorders.

Atypical Affective Disorders include Atypical Bipolar and Atypical Depression, disorders that cannot be classified in either the Major Affective or Other Specific Affective Disorders class.

A diagnosis of Affective Disorder can be considered when the mood disturbance is primary and central, not secondary to some other disorder. When the cause of the mood disturbance is known to be organicity or Schizophrenia, these diagnoses take precedence. When the mood disturbance is a mild one stemming from psychosocial stress, the diagnosis of Adjustment Disorder takes precedence.

DEPRESSIVE AND MANIC SYNDROMES

The two building blocks of Affective Disorders are the depressive syndrome and the manic syndrome. Each syndrome has at its core the disordered mood; the remainder of the syndrome is a set of associated features. Both of these syndromes are clinical clusters of symptoms that might be produced by a number of causes.

Depressive Syndrome

The features of the depressive syndrome can be grouped in four areas: mood, vitality, agitation, and consolation-seeking behavior. Mood is the core of this syndrome. The pervasive influence of mood is evident in the associated features.

Features of Depression

Mood

Sadness—gloominess, tearfulness, dejection, devastation.

Demoralization—loss of enthusiasm, loss of humor, loss of values in goals, death wishes.

Ennui—boredom, lack of interest in new things, loss of old interests, loss of interest in friends.

Self-derogation—feeling messed up, inferior, to blame, no good, worthless.

Vitality

Well-being—feeling "off," not well, listless, mentally dull, unable to think.

Stamina—trouble getting started, mopey, draggy, washed out, tired, falling behind.

Appetite—loss of zest for eating, lack of hunger, weight loss, trouble eating.

Libido—avoidance, absence of enjoyment, absence of desire.

Agitation

Anxiety—apprehension, dread, tension, somatization, anguish, panic.

Turmoil—brooding, fretfulness, worry, irritability.

Sleep—delayed, shallow, unrefreshing, interrupted, nightmares.

Behavior—restless, fidgety, chain-smoking, nail-biting, wasteful spending, reckless risks, self-destructive acts.

Consolation-Seeking Behavior

Relationships—clinging, demanding, pleading, occasionally hypersexuality.

Escape—withdrawal into solitude, taking to bed, excess sleep.

Food, Drugs, Alcohol—excessive reliance, excessive intake, weight gain.

Manic Syndrome

71   The manic syndrome is at the other end of the continuum—perhaps more enjoyable but just as deranged. The features of mania can be grouped in four areas: mood, vitality, agitation, and pleasure-seeking behavior.

Features of Mania

Mood

Elation—cheerfulness, high spirits.

Humor—joking, clowning, irrepressible infectious quality.

Schemes—into everything, flighty, distractible.

Expansiveness—feeling unusually gifted, superior, talented.

Vitality

Well-being—feeling robust, exuberant, on top of the world.

Stamina—tireless, refreshed with minimum sleep.

Appetite—zest for eating, tendency to excess.

Libido—enhanced, interest expressed readily, possibly promiscuous.

Agitation

Turmoil—may have urgent sense of restlessness.

Irritability—may be demanding, pushy, especially when curbed.

Behavior—restless, constant motion, loud speech, possibly somewhat physically aggressive.

Pleasure-Seeking Behavior

Relationships—unnatural warmth, engages strangers, may show undue generosity, may be on the phone into the middle of the night.

Food, Drugs, Alcohol—indiscretion and excesses.

CLASSIFICATION OF AFFECTIVE DISORDERS

2 The mood syndromes are on a continuum with the normal mood range as illustrated in Table 10. The normal ups and downs of mood are within zone one; moving beyond that into zone two represents a partial depressive or manic syndrome; moving all the way into zone three represents a full-blown depressive or manic syndrome. A partial manic syndrome is also called "hypomania"; a partial depressive syndrome could be called "mild depression."

3 The presence of a full or partial manic or depressive syndrome is one component in the diagnosis of an Affective Disorder. Other components to consider in making the diagnosis are the presence of highs and lows and the duration of the syndrome.

Examination of the individual's history is important in classifying Affective Disorders. If there have been any highs (either alone or intermixed with lows), the disorder will fall into the Bipolar Group. If there have been only lows and no highs, the disorder will fall into the Unipolar Depressive Groups.

The reason for classifying even an isolated high as Bipolar is that there is evidence from research to presume that there will eventually be some lows, and the genetic and treatment response data suggest that "unipolar mania" is a Bipolar Disorder.

Table 11 represents the reasoning in the classification. A history of the presence of highs and/or lows places the disorder in the correct column. The next step, which places it in the correct row, is determining the duration and extent of the mood disturbance: full syndrome, partial chronic syndrome, or an atypical syndrome which does not quite fit the two above.

74 Table 12 is a graphic illustration of Table 11. The alignment is the same, a column of disorders that have highs, either alone or intermixed with lows,

TABLE 10
Continuum of Mood Syndromes

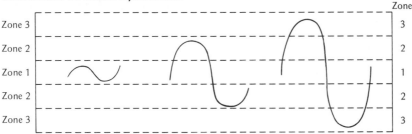

TABLE 11
Classification of Affective Disorders

Syndrome	Bipolar Group	Unipolar Depressive Group
Full Syndrome, Major Affective Disorders	Bipolar Disorder	Major Depression
Chronic Partial Syndrome, Other Specific Affective Disorders	Cyclothymic Disorder	Dysthymic Disorder
Atypical Syndrome	Atypical Bipolar Disorder	Atypical Depression

and a column of disorders that have only lows and no highs. As in the previous mood graphs, zone one represents normal mood; zone two is for partial syndrome; and zone three is full syndrome. Points above zone one represent manic episodes, and those below represent depressive episodes.

Bipolar Group
The Bipolar Group includes disorders where there is evidence of a manic or hypomanic episode. It includes Bipolar Disorder, Cyclothymic Disorder, and Atypical Bipolar Disorder.

Bipolar Disorder (zone three) represents the full syndrome of the Bipolar Group. The individual may be seen at a point when she/he is manic, depressed, or mixed (a coexistence of manic and depressive syndromes at the *same* time). However, if the full manic syndrome is reached at any one time in the individual's history, the diagnosis of Bipolar Disorder is made and will remain the diagnosis even if subsequent recurrences are milder.

A Cyclothymic Disorder is diagnosed if the full manic syndrome is not reached (lines remain in zone two—hypomania and mild depression) and the condition continues for a period of time.

Atypical Bipolar Disorder does not fit the pattern for Bipolar or Cyclothymic Disorders (i.e., single hypomanic episode; hypomanic episode followed by full depressive syndrome; conditions with highs that don't fit the criteria for Bipolar and Cyclothymic Disorder).

Unipolar Depressive Group

The Unipolar Depressive Group includes disorders where there are only lows: Major Depression, Dysthymic Disorder, and Atypical Depression.

Major Depression is a disorder composed of only the full depressive syndrome (lines in zone three) and can be recurrent or single episode.

Dysthymic Disorder is diagnosed when there is a chronic partial pattern (lines in zone two) with at least two years of steady mild depression, with normal mood for only short intervals.

Atypical Depression is a diagnosis used for conditions without highs that do not fit the criteria for Major Depression or Dysthymic Disorder (i.e., a single short episode of mild depression; recurrent short depressive episodes with long periods of normal mood).

TABLE 12
Classification of Syndromes

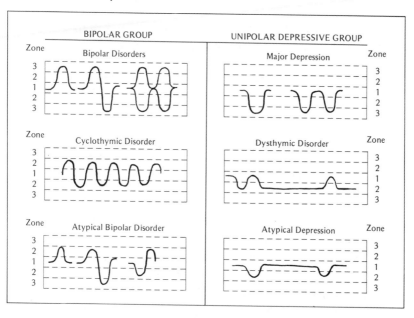

Another example of Atypical Depression could be a case of Schizophrenia, Residual Type, where a full depressive syndrome develops following recovery from the acute psychotic phase or without activation of the psychotic symptoms.

DIAGNOSTIC CRITERIA—BIPOLAR GROUP

For a diagnosis of Bipolar Disorder to be made, there first must be a manic episode, either currently or in the past. The diagnostic criteria for a manic episode are as follows:

75

(1) Distinct periods with prominent and relatively persistent elevated or irritable mood.

(2) Duration of at least a week or requiring hospitalization.

(3) At least three of the symptoms listed in DSM-III, p. 208, (four, if the mood is only irritable).

(4) Rule out Schizophrenia, related psychoses, organicity.

This list of symptoms is a guide to qualify as a full manic episode. If the quota is not met, then only a partial syndrome exists (hypomania), and a Bipolar Disorder would not be diagnosed.

Bipolar Disorder

76   Bipolar Disorder needs to be subclassified as to the nature of the current episode at the fourth digit as: Manic, Depressed, or Mixed.

Bipolar Disorder, Manic is diagnosed when an individual, either currently or recently, meets the previously stated criteria for a manic episode. If a person has experienced a manic episode in the past, it is not necessary that the present episode meet the full criteria.

Bipolar Disorder, Depressed is diagnosed when a person has had *one or more manic episodes* and the current or recent clinical picture is characterized by a major depressive episode that meets the following diagnostic criteria:

77

(1) Prominent and persistent dysphoric mood.

(2) Duration of at least two weeks.

(3) At least four of the symptoms listed in DSM-III, p. 214. (For children under six, at least three of the first four.)

(4) Not superimposed on Schizophrenia or related psychoses.

(5) Not due to any Organic Disorder or Uncomplicated Bereavement.

The list of symptoms is a guide to qualify this as a *full* depressive episode; if the quota is not met, then only a partial syndrome exists.

Bipolar Disorder, Mixed is diagnosed when there is a full symptomatic range of manic as well as major depressive aspects in the current clinical picture. The depressive symptoms must be prominent and exist for at least one day.

Cyclothymic Disorder

Cyclothymic Disorder, also in the bipolar group, is characterized by symptoms of both the manic and depressive syndromes. However, the symptoms are not of sufficient severity or duration to be classified as a major depressive or manic episode. This condition was previously called "cyclothymic personality."

This is a familial condition on a continuum with Bipolar Disorder and can intensify into Bipolar Disorder.

Diagnostic criteria for Cyclothymic Disorder include:

(1) at least two years of alternation between mild manic and depressive syndromes that do not reach the extent of a Major Affective Disorder.

(2) at least three of the DSM-III symptoms listed on p. 220 for mild depressive and manic syndromes.

(3) no psychotic features.

(4) not secondary to any other mental disorder.

If this disorder does intensify into a Major Affective Disorder, the diagnosis will be changed.

Atypical Bipolar Disorder

Atypical Bipolar Disorder must have some manic features, yet not quite meet the criteria for Bipolar or Cyclothymic Disorders. A single hypomanic episode would be called Atypical Bipolar Disorder.

DIAGNOSTIC CRITERIA—UNIPOLAR GROUP

Major Depression

Major Depression is the most severe disorder in the Unipolar Depressive Group. (The commonality of the Unipolar Depressive Group is that there are lows without any highs.)

The criteria for Major Depression are the same as those of the depressive episode of the Bipolar Disorders. What distinguishes Major Depression from the Bipolar Disorders is the fact that for a Major Depression there must not be evidence of a manic episode. Other diagnostic criteria include:

(1) prominent and persistent dysphoric mood.

(2) duration of at least two weeks.

(3) at least four symptoms listed in DSM-III, p. 214. (For children under six, at least three of the first four.)

(4) not superimposed on Schizophrenia or related psychoses.

(5) not due to any Organic Disorder or uncomplicated bereavement.

For Major Depression the distinction must be made as to whether the depression is a single episode or a recurrent condition. This distinction is indicated by a fourth digit code.

Dysthymic Disorder

80 Dysthymic Disorder, also in the Unipolar Depressive Group, requires two years or more of fairly steady mild depressive symptoms. The diagnostic criteria include:

(1) at least two years (one year for children and adolescents) of mild depressive symptoms that do not reach the extent of Major Depression.

(2) short periods of normal mood may intervene.

(3) at least three of the listed mild depressive symptoms.

(4) not simply a set of depressive symptoms that are part of another Axis I disorder.

If this condition worsens to the magnitude of Major Depression, that diagnosis must be added.

Atypical Depression

Atypical Depression is a set of Affective Disorders in the Unipolar Depressive Group that do not meet the criteria for Major Depression or Dysthymic Disorder.

There are no specific diagnostic criteria for this disorder. Examples include:

(1) mild depressions that are not chronic (i.e., have not existed for a period of two years or more).

(2) mild depressions interspersed with long periods of normal moods.

(3) mild depressions that are not clearly in response to a recent stressor, thus ruling out Adjustment Disorder.

(4) other unusual depressions.

FIFTH DIGIT CODING

81 **Bipolar Disorder, Manic** and **Bipolar Disorder, Mixed** are similarly defined in the fifth digit according to the associated features:

- *without psychotic features*
- *with mood-congruent psychotic features*
- *with mood-incongruent psychotic features*
- *in remission*

Mood-congruent psychotic features are consistent with the elevated mood (a delusion that one is Howard Hughes' heir, for example). Psychotic features may develop that are not consistent with the elevated mood (a delusion that has a bizarre quality, for example) and would be considered mood-incongruent.

82 **Bipolar Disorder, Depressed** is coded in the fifth digit according to associated features:

- *without melancholia*
- *with melancholia*
- *with mood-congruent psychotic features*
- *with mood-incongruent psychotic features*
- *in remission*

By the time there is melancholia in the picture, there are endogenous features and the individual may be absorbed, out of reach, and unresponsive to environmental changes.

An example of a mood-congruent delusion is an individual who feels that he/she is a terrible sinner and should be exterminated. A mood-incongruent delusion might be a bizarre delusion unrelated to the down or depressed mood.

Cyclothymic Disorder, Dysthymic Disorder, Atypical Depression, and **Atypical Bipolar Disorder** do not use fifth digit codes.

CASE VIGNETTE

Harold, a 27-year-old Coca-cola truck driver, functioned in a routine manner until three weeks ago when his wife suffered a miscarriage. He was found shortly afterward to be in surprisingly and increasingly high spirits—talking loudly and animatedly, clowning around, and cracking jokes that became increasingly crude and coarse. Co-workers, who found this amusing at first, found it exhausting after a while, and they complained that he was racing through his work in a reckless fashion. Warned that his job was in jeopardy, he declared that he didn't need it anymore since he had just invented a new drink that would outsell Coca-cola and make him a billionaire. A friend from the lab analyzed the drink and found it to be no more than club soda with vanilla flavoring. Undaunted, Harold claimed that this wonder drink would also be a cancer cure that would bring him the Nobel Prize.

Somehow, Harold talked the neighborhood bank into a $10,000 loan for his venture, but the family soon found that he had given considerable amounts to strangers, whom he referred to as "business associates," after meeting them in bars. He had been spending most of his nights in bars, since he was tireless despite only two or three hours of sleep a night. The family finally persuaded him to come into the hospital.

When the doctor arrived, Harold bounded over and greeted him in an effusive warm manner, as if they were old buddies, and made several grand, cavalier-like gestures in a ceremonial fashion, as if this were a gala occasion. Harold's voice and manner were irrepressively humorous; on hearing the doctor's name, he spun off seven puns in rapid succession associated with the name.

Discussion Guide

The Decision Tree for Differential Diagnosis of Mood Disturbance, DSM-III, p. 344, may be useful in this discussion.

In diagnosing this case, note the time frame, the primary disturbance in mood, the features of mania, and the distinction of mood-congruent psychotic features.

The differential diagnosis should be reviewed to rule out Organic Mental Disorders and Schizophrenia or Schizoaffective Disorder.

83   **Answer**—See Answers, Chapter 12.

Chapter 13

Anxiety Disorders

GENERAL OVERVIEW

Many of the conditions formerly labeled "neurosis" are now under the heading of Anxiety Disorders. A few are included in Dissociative, Somatoform, and Psychosexual Disorders. The condition previously known as "neurotic depression" is classified in DSM-III as an Affective Disorder.

Anxiety is the central feature in this group of disorders. Anxiety is either the predominant disturbance or experienced if an individual attempts to master or resist certain specific symptoms (e.g., phobic objects or compulsive rituals).

The basic features of anxiety as described in DSM-III are:

(1) Motor tension demonstrated by being jumpy, trembling, or unable to relax.

(2) Autonomic hyperactivity evidenced by dizziness, racing heart, or perspiring.

(3) Apprehensive expectation demonstrated by anxious rumination.

(4) Vigilance and scanning evidenced by hyperattentiveness.

In DSM-II anxiety was the signal of neurosis. All disorders in which anxiety was "felt and expressed directly" or "controlled unconsciously" by conversion, displacement, and other defense mechanisms were classified as "neuroses." In DSM-III only disorders in which anxiety is experienced directly are included in the class of Anxiety Disorders.

Diagnosis in this class of disorders follows a hierarchical system with more specific classes of diagnosis taking precedence over more general classes.

93

In other words, an individual with phobic features and generalized anxiety would be given a Phobic Disorder diagnosis rather than a Generalized Anxiety Disorder diagnosis.

85   The following are subclasses of the Anxiety Disorders: Phobic, Obsessive Compulsive, Panic, Generalized Anxiety, Post-traumatic Stress, and Atypical Anxiety. With Phobic and Obsessive Compulsive Disorders, anxiety is experienced if an individual resists giving into his/her symptoms. Anxiety is the predominant disturbance in an individual with Panic, Generalized Anxiety, or Post-traumatic Stress Disorders.

PHOBIC DISORDERS

86   Phobic Disorders are the most specific subclass of the Anxiety Disorders and include: Agoraphobia, with and without panic attacks, Social Phobia, and Simple Phobia.

The essential features of all the Phobic Disorders are:

(1) Persistent avoidance behavior secondary to irrational fears.

(2) Recognition of the fear as unreasonable and unwarranted.

(3) Avoidance behavior and fear causing subjective distress or interfering with social or role functioning.

The various types of Phobic Disorders differ in their clinical picture, characteristic age of onset, and their differential treatment response (Marks, 1968).

In DSM-II, all the phobias were classified as "phobic neurosis."

87   **Agoraphobia** is characterized by a marked fear and avoidance of being alone or in public places. There is also an increasing restriction of normal activities. In the diagnosis of Agoraphobia, the presence or absence of panic attacks is noted in the history.

If a phobic avoidance of certain situations is due to another disorder, such as Paranoid Personality Disorder or Major Depression, the diagnosis of Agoraphobia is not made. An individual who stays at home because Martians are after him is not an agoraphobic! The same is true of all the Phobic Disorders.

88   **Social Phobia** has as its essential feature a persistent, irrational fear and a compelling desire to avoid situations where the individual may be exposed to the scrutiny of others. Individuals with Social Phobia are distressed by this disturbance and recognize its excessiveness. Social Phobias are not due to

other mental disorders. Examples of Social Phobia are fear and avoidance of speaking in public, eating in public, using public lavatories. These phobias are *not* to be confused with normal fear or apprehension in such settings.

Simple Phobia is a residual category for specific phobias which are not Agoraphobia or Social Phobias. A Simple Phobia is a fear and avoidance of an object or situation such as animals or heights. A person with a Simple Phobia is distressed by this disturbance and recognizes its unreasonableness. Once again, the fear and avoidance must not be due to another mental disorder.

OBSESSIVE COMPULSIVE DISORDER

The essential elements of the Obsessive Compulsive Disorder are recurrent obsessions and/or compulsions. Obsessions are recurrent, persistent ideas, thoughts, images, or impulses that are experienced as being senseless, repugnant, and involuntarily produced. Compulsions are repetitive and seemingly purposeful behaviors that are performed according to certain rules or in stereotyped fashion. They are designed to produce or prevent some future event or situation.

Obsessive Compulsive Disorder may feature either obsessions or compulsions or both. The disorder is a source of distress and interferes with an individual's role or function. The symptoms must not be due to another mental disorder.

Compulsive behaviors must be distinguished from conditions known as Disorders of Impulse Control Not Elsewhere Classified when there is a sense of pleasure or release while committing the act (e.g., Pathological Gambling).

In DSM-II, this disorder was called "obsessive compulsive neurosis."

PANIC DISORDER

The condition identified as "anxiety neurosis" in DSM-II is conceptualized in DSM-III as two separate disorders: Panic Disorder and Generalized Anxiety Disorder. The essential features of a Panic Disorder are recurrent panic attacks marked by the sudden onset of intense apprehension, fear or terror, and often accompanied by feelings of impending doom.

The diagnostic criteria for Panic Disorder include: three panic attacks in three weeks in non-life-threatening circumstances; discrete periods of apprehension; and four of 12 symptoms outlined in DSM-III, p. 231.

Panic Disorder is not due to another mental or physical disorder and is not associated with Agoraphobia.

There is some evidence that a Panic Disorder has a differential treatment

response when compared to other Anxiety Disorders where anxiety is prominent (Klein et al., 1978; Zitrin et al., 1978).

GENERALIZED ANXIETY DISORDER

The basic element of the Generalized Anxiety Disorder is persistent anxiety of
at least one month's duration without specific symptoms as in Phobic or Obsessive Compulsive Disorders.

92   The diagnostic criteria for this disorder include generalized, persistent
anxiety, with symptoms from three of four characteristic features of anxiety
discussed at the opening of this chapter. It also includes an anxious mood
continuous for one month and is not due to another mental disorder. To re-
ceive this diagnosis, the individual must be 18 years or older.

When making this diagnosis, it is important to rule out physical disorders (e.g., hyperthyroidism), Organic Mental Disorders (e.g., caffeine intoxication), and other mental disorders.

POST-TRAUMATIC STRESS DISORDER

93   The essential feature of Post-traumatic Stress Disorder is the development of
certain symptoms, following a psychologically traumatic event that is outside the range of usual human experiences. It is almost the equivalent of psychological "shock." Examples of traumatic events are rape, earthquakes, being held hostage, and the Vietnam war.

In DSM-II, this condition was called "traumatic neurosis."

To diagnose this disorder, there must exist a stressor and a numbing of
responses to, or reduced involvement with, the external world. There is also a
reexperiencing of the trauma in one of three ways, and the development of
two of six symptoms that were not pre-trauma, as outlined in DSM-III, p.
238.

94   Depending on the temporal relationship of the symptom to the trauma,
this condition can be either acute, delayed, or chronic. If symptoms occur
within six months of the trauma, it is considered *acute*. If the onset occurs at
least six months after the trauma, the condition is labeled *delayed*. When the
symptoms last for more than six months, it would be considered *chronic*.

Post-traumatic Stress Disorder must be differentiated from an Adjustment Disorder where the stressor and reaction are less severe. If Anxiety, Affective, or Organic Disorders develop, these diagnoses should also be made.

ATYPICAL ANXIETY DISORDER

This diagnosis should be used when the clinician cannot be more specific.

CASE VIGNETTE

Harry is a 40-year-old white male who comes to intake because he is feeling very nervous. During the past month he has been overwhelmed by anxiety on at least eight to ten different occasions. These "fits" come on suddenly and happen at work, at home, and sometimes while he is driving. He gets dizzy, begins to sweat, and becomes very tense. The attacks scare him because he feels he is going to lose all control. He has no history of mental problems and this is the first time he has come to a clinic for help. He has been to his medical doctors but they could not find anything physically wrong. At first, he thought he might be having a heart attack. Harry does not know why these attacks occur and wants to get rid of them.

Discussion Guide

To assist in the diagnosis of Anxiety Disorders use the Decision Tree for Differential Diagnosis of Irrational Anxiety and Avoidance Behavior, DSM-III, pp. 342–343.

In this case there are distinct, recurrent anxiety attacks which meet the criteria for a Panic Disorder. These attacks occur in a wide variety of situations and have not caused the individual to avoid certain situations which would be required for an Agoraphobia diagnosis. Physical causes are ruled out first with a medical exam. Only if the anxiety were persistent and not in the form of discrete attacks, could the diagnosis of Generalized Anxiety Disorder be considered.

Answer—See Answers, Chapter 13.

Chapter 14

Somatoform Disorders

GENERAL OVERVIEW

Conditions in this group of disorders present in the form of somatic complaints. However, symptoms suggesting physical illness can be classified under various categories in DSM-III. These include: Somatoform Disorders, Factitious Disorders, Malingering, and Psychological Factors Affecting Physical Condition. In addition to these categories, physical symptoms could also represent an undiagnosed physical illness.

The essential features of Somatoform Disorders include:

96

(1) Physical symptoms which suggest a physical disorder.

(2) No demonstrable organic findings or known physiological mechanisms.

(3) Evidence or presumption that the symptoms are associated with psychological factors.

(4) Symptoms not voluntarily controlled.

Clinical judgment is needed in assessing the degree of control the individual has over the symptoms and their relationship to psychological factors.

A child's stomachache on the morning of a test at school would not be a Somatoform Disorder! It would probably be classified as Malingering, as there is a recognizable environmental goal.

DSM-III has brought together in this category a number of diagnoses which were under various DSM-II categories like "hysterical neurosis, conversion type," and "hypochondriacal neurosis."

The types or subclasses in this group are Somatization Disorder, Conversion Disorder, Psychogenic Pain Disorder, Hypochondriasis, and Atypical Somatoform Disorder.

SOMATIZATION DISORDER

The clinical picture in Somatization Disorder features recurrent and multiple somatic complaints of several years' duration, beginning before the age of 30.

Somatic complaints after the age of 30 are almost always attributable to a physical condition or interpreted by the individual to represent a definite physical illness. In this case a diagnosis of Hypochondriasis should be considered.

The number of complaints in the diagnostic criteria differ according to the gender of the individual. To meet this criteria, 14 of 37 symptoms are required for women and 12 of 37 for men. This is not a sexist distinction, but is needed because one of the general classes of symptoms focuses on menstrual problems or complaints. A complete listing of the types of complaints or symptoms needed for this diagnosis can be found in DSM-III, pp. 243–244. It is very important to rule out physical disorders, as well as somatic delusions, in making this diagnosis.

Dysthymic Disorder and Generalized Anxiety Disorder are not diagnosed in individuals who are depressed or anxious as a result of the multiple somatic complaints of their Somatization Disorder.

In DSM-II, this condition was referred to as "hysteria," and elsewhere in the literature was called Briquet's Syndrome.

CONVERSION DISORDER

The term "Conversion Disorder" was developed with the implication that there is a specific mechanism to account for the disturbance. DSM-III continues to take this perspective, and considers that either primary or secondary gain are operating in the development of this disorder.

Primary gain is the mechanism whereby the individual keeps an internal conflict or need out of his/her awareness, such as a paralysis of the arm reflecting a conflict about the expression of rage. Secondary gain is the mechanism whereby the individual manages to avoid a particularly noxious activity or gets support from the environment not otherwise forthcoming. A paralyzed hand that makes it impossible for a soldier to fire a gun is an example of this.

The predominant disturbance of a Conversion Disorder is a loss of or alteration in physical functioning that suggests a physical disorder but apparently expresses a psychological conflict or need.

The symptoms must not be under voluntary control. Otherwise, a Factitious Disorder or Malingering would need to be considered. In addition, the symptoms are not limited problems of pain or sexual dysfunction, nor are they part of a Somatization Disorder or Schizophrenia.

There is no physical or pathophysiological explanation for the complaint. The symptoms usually appear suddenly and often there is a lack of concern about the symptoms.

The Conversion Disorder can also be called Hysterical Neurosis, Conversion Type.

PSYCHOGENIC PAIN DISORDER

99   If the predominant problem of an individual is the complaint of pain in the absence of adequate physical explanations and with evidence of associated psychological factors, then the diagnosis of Psychogenic Pain Disorder should be made.

The pain must be either inconsistent with neurological and pathological findings or be an abnormal level of pain for any existing physical condition, and not be due to another mental disorder. Pain associated with tension headaches is not diagnosed as Psychogenic Pain Disorder, since there is a physiologic mechanism that accounts for the pain.

This is a new category and careful assessment is needed to make this diagnosis.

HYPOCHONDRIASIS

100   If the predominant disturbance is an unrealistic interpretation that physical signs or sensations are abnormal, leading to a fear or belief of having a serious disease, then the condition would be diagnosed as Hypochondriasis. The preoccupation may be with bodily functions or with a specific organ or single disease. The belief interferes with normal functioning despite medical reassurance, and is not due to another disorder. Fear of the disease would be more predominant than multiple somatic complaints which would be diagnosed as a Somatization Disorder.

ATYPICAL SOMATOFORM DISORDER

This is a leftover category to be used when the condition meets the general criteria for a Somatoform Disorder but the clinician cannot be more specific.

CASE VIGNETTE

Aretha is a 37-year-old secretary who is currently separated from her husband. Five months ago she discovered that her husband was having an affair and he then asked for a divorce. Six weeks ago she began coughing and having a difficult time breathing. She went to her doctor but he could find nothing wrong. However, she was not convinced of his findings. She believes that she has lung cancer. Her father died of lung cancer five years ago and Aretha has smoked cigarettes since she was 14. She is also losing weight, which she feels confirms her belief. She has gone to cancer specialists and had x-rays which were negative. However, no one has been able to explain her persistent coughing and she remains convinced that she has lung cancer. Recently she lost her job because she has taken off so many sick days for doctor's visits and because she stays home in bed.

Discussion Guide

The Decision Tree for Differential Diagnosis of Physical Complaints and Irrational Anxiety about Physical Illness, DSM-III, pp. 346–347, can be utilized in reviewing this case.

The critical element in arriving at this diagnosis is the belief of serious disease despite disconfirming medical evidence. This belief is causing occupational dysfunction and psychological factors are judged to be relevant.

Answer—See Answers, Chapter 14.

Chapter 15

Dissociative Disorders

GENERAL OVERVIEW
The class of Dissociative Disorders has the following basic features:

102
(1) A sudden temporary alteration in the normally integrated functions of consciousness, identity or motor behavior.

(2) Some part of one or more functions is lost.

(3) This alteration or loss of function is not due to organic causes.

Although a Sleepwalking Disorder involves dissociation, it is classified in DSM-III as a Disorder Usually First Evident in Infancy, Childhood, or Adolescence.

It is important to rule out Organic Mental Disorders, including any dissociated states caused by drugs or alcohol.

In DSM-II these disorders were classified as "hysterical neurosis, dissociative types."

103
The subclasses of Dissociative Disorders are Psychogenic Amnesia, Psychogenic Fugue, Multiple Personality, Depersonalization Disorder, and what has now become a typical category, the Atypical Dissociative Disorder.

PSYCHOGENIC AMNESIA
To be given a diagnosis of Psychogenic Amnesia, the condition must be characterized by sudden inability, not due to an Organic Mental Disorder, to recall important personal information. The deficit in recall must also be too great to be explained by ordinary forgetfulness (I forgot!!).

The disturbance in recall can be *localized or circumscribed amnesia.*

This is a failure to recall events in a circumscribed period of time. It can also be *selective amnesia*—a failure to recall some but not all events during a period of time. Failure to recall the individual's entire life is *generalized amnesia*, and *continuous amnesia* is a failure to recall events subsequent to a specific time and up to and including the present.

Since memory impairment is often associated with organic conditions, it is extremely important to rule out Organic Mental Disorders when making the diagnosis of Psychogenic Amnesia.

PSYCHOGENIC FUGUE

Fugue means flight, and the predominant features of Psychogenic Fugue are sudden, unexpected travel away from home or work locale with the assumption of a new identity and an inability to recall the previous identity. Wandering can also appear in Psychogenic Amnesia, but it is more purposeful in a Psychogenic Fugue.

Again, it is important to rule out Organic Mental Disorders when making this diagnosis.

MULTIPLE PERSONALITY

The predominant presenting symptom in the diagnosis of Multiple Personality is the existence of two or more distinct personalities in one individual. Each personality is an integrated unit with its own memories, behaviors, and relationships, and becomes the dominant and controlling force in the individual's life at a particular time. Subpersonalities are often not aware of each other and the shift from one to another generally occurs under stress and quite suddenly.

Although the disorder is rare, the dramatic nature of the disorder has made it a popular one in the literature (e.g., Sybil, Three Faces of Eve). This disorder is not diagnosed in individuals who simply report that they feel like two different people at times or when hallucinations or delusions are responsible for what seem to be other personalities.

DEPERSONALIZATION DISORDER

In the diagnosis of a Depersonalization Disorder, the predominant disturbance is one or more episodes of depersonalization causing impairment in social or occupational functioning. The experience of depersonalization includes a sense of estrangement from the normal sense of self, feelings of unreality, dream-like states, and, at times, bodily sensations that are strange and ego-dystonic. Reality-testing, however, remains intact.

Onset of this disorder after the age of 40 is rare. Mild depersonalization experiences often occur in young adults when their sense of self is not solidly established. However, if these experiences do not produce significant impairment, they are not diagnosed as a Depersonalization Disorder.

ATYPICAL DISSOCIATIVE DISORDER

This is an additional category that includes dissociated states in persons who may have undergone intense coercive persuasion (e.g., brainwashing, indoctrination). The defense's assertion in the Patty Hearst trial that "Tanya" was a dissociated state, produced by her captivity, would be classified as an Atypical Dissociative Disorder.

CASE VIGNETTE

Burt Tate is a 42-year-old white male. He was brought to the emergency room by the police. He had been in a fight in the diner where he worked. When the police began to question him, they discovered that he had no identification, that he had drifted into town last week and begun working as a short-order cook at the diner. He did not know where he had come from before this time and could not recall any details of his past life. When the police ran a description check on him, they found that he fit the description of Gene Smith, a missing person who disappeared one month ago from a town 200 miles away. A physical exam did not uncover any head trauma and there was no evidence of drug abuse. A visit by his wife confirmed the real identity of the man as Gene Smith. His wife explained that he had been having a lot of problems with his job and had been under a considerable amount of stress. There was no history of any previous psychiatric disorder or serious medical problem.

Discussion Guide

In this case there is the loss of memory of a previous identity and the assumption of a new one. The central feature is the flight to another town, the hallmark of Psychogenic Fugue. Note the psychosocial stress related to the flight.

Answer—See Answers, Chapter 15.

Chapter 16

Psychosexual Disorders

GENERAL OVERVIEW
The diagnostic class of Psychosexual Disorders includes disorders of sexual identity, functioning, and dysfunction in which psychological factors are assumed to play a major role.

Sexual functioning problems exclusively caused by organic factors are not diagnosed in this class of disorders. The organic cause should appear on Axis III. If psychological factors also interact with the physical disorder, a diagnosis of Psychological Factors Affecting Physical Condition or one of the Adjustment Disorders would be made on Axis I.

There are four subclasses of Psychosexual Disorders: Gender Identity Disorders, Paraphilias, Psychosexual Dysfunctions, and Other Psychosexual Disorders. In the field trials, this group of disorders demonstrated very good interrater agreement because they are very distinguishable categories with clear and concise diagnostic criteria.

Psychosexual Disorders in DSM-III include a number of different terms and categories not included in DSM-II.

GENDER IDENTITY DISORDERS
The central problem in the Gender Identity Disorders is a conflict or incongruence between the actual, anatomical sex of an individual and the gender identity or inner sense of gender.

The three groups of Gender Identity Disorders are Transsexualism, Gender Identity Disorder of Childhood, and Atypical Gender Identity Disorder. These disorders are rare and are not to be confused with unhappiness with one's sexual role or fears of inadequacy about living up to the expectations of that role.

Transsexualism should be diagnosed when a person has had a persistent and continuous (for at least two years) sense of discomfort and inappropriateness regarding his/her anatomical sex, and a desire to be rid of his/her genitals and live as a member of the opposite sex.

Transsexualism should not be diagnosed when there is a genetic abnormality or the presence of abnormal sexual structural characteristics, nor when the identity disorder is due to another mental disorder.

The sexual history of an individual with the diagnosis of Transsexualism is noted in the 5th digit as: 1—*asexual*, 2—*homosexual*, 3—*heterosexual*, or 0—*unspecified*.

Note the difference between Transsexualism as a Gender Identity Disorder and Transvestism under Paraphilias.

Gender Identity Disorder of Childhood consists of persistent discomfort and a sense of inappropriateness about a child's anatomical sex and the desire to be, or insistence that he/she is, of the other sex. The onset of this disorder must be before puberty and includes a repudiation of the individual's own anatomical attributes or, for boys, preoccupation with stereotypical female activities.

Atypical Gender Identity Disorder is a residual category. This diagnosis should be used for adults who have features similar to the Gender Identity Disorder of Childhood or for any other gender identity disturbance not more specifically classifiable.

PARAPHILIAS

107   The "sexual deviations" that appeared in DSM-II are now referred to as Paraphilias. This new term emphasizes the unusual or bizarre acts or imagery (para) to which the individual is attracted (philia).

Paraphilias involve: the use of nonliving objects or fetishes as a method of achieving sexual excitement; repeated sexual activities with human partners that involve real or simulated suffering or humiliation; or repeated sexual activity with nonconsenting partners. The disorder should be diagnosed only if the bizarre imagery or acts become necessary or preferred for sexual excitement or release of sexual and non-erotic tension.

Fetishism refers to the use of nonliving objects or fetishes as an exclusive or preferred way of becoming sexually excited. Fetishes are not limited to clothing or objects designed for sexual stimulation, such as a vibrator.

Transvestism is a recurrent and persistent cross-dressing, or dressing like a woman, by a heterosexual male. In the initial course of the disorder, cross-dressing is used for the purpose of sexual excitement. There is intense frustration when the cross-dressing is interfered with.

Transvestism does not meet the criteria for Transsexualism.

Zoophilia involves acts or fantasies of engaging in sexual activity with animals as a repeatedly preferred or exclusive method of achieving sexual excitement.

Pedophilia involves acts or fantasies of engaging in sexual activity with prepubertal children as a repeatedly preferred or exclusive method of achieving sexual excitement.

Exhibitionism is the repetitive act of exposing the genitals to an unsuspecting stranger for the purpose of achieving sexual excitement, with no attempt at further sexual activity with the stranger.

Voyeurism refers to an individual who repeatedly observes unsuspecting people who are naked, in the act of disrobing, or engaging in sexual activity. No sexual activity with the observed people is sought. Such observations are the repeatedly preferred or exclusive methods of achieving sexual excitement.

Sexual Masochism is a preferred or exclusive mode of producing sexual excitement by being humiliated, bound, beaten or otherwise made to suffer. The individual has intentionally participated in an activity in which he/she was physically harmed or his/her life was threatened, in order to produce sexual excitement.

Sexual Sadism involving a nonconsenting partner occurs when the disordered individual has repeatedly and intentionally inflicted psychological or physical suffering in order to produce sexual excitement. With a consenting partner, the repeatedly preferred or exclusive mode of achieving sexual excitement combines humiliation with simulated or mildly injurious bodily suffering. Also with a consenting partner, bodily injury that is extensive, permanent, or possibly mortal is inflicted in order to achieve sexual excitement.

Atypical Paraphilia includes: Coprophilia (feces); Frotteurism (rubbing); Klismaphilia (enema); Mysophilia (filth); Necrophilia (corpse); Telephone Scatologia (lewdness); and Urophilia (urine).

PSYCHOSEXUAL DYSFUNCTIONS
108   Psychosexual Dysfunctions are disturbances in the desire or psychophysiological responses that characterize the four phases of the sexual response cycle.

The *Desire* or *Appetitive Phase* consists of fantasies about sexual activity and a desire to have sexual activity. The *Excitement Phase* consists of a subjective sense of sexual pleasure and accompanying physiological changes. The *Orgasm Phase* consists of a peaking of sexual pleasure, with release of sexual tension and rhythmic contraction of the perineal muscles and pelvic reproductive organs. The *Resolution Phase* consists of a sense of general relaxation, well-being, and muscular relaxation. In DSM-III, there are no disorders related to this phase of sexual functioning.

This is a new category based on the research and conceptualization of the sexual response cycle from the works of Kaplan (1979), Masters and Johnson (1970), and others.

In making a diagnosis from this class it is important to first establish if the dysfunction is due to organic factors, medication use, or another Axis I diagnosis. If the dysfunction is a result of medication, a physical injury or illness such as a spinal cord injury or diabetes, or a preceding depression, the problem is not diagnosed as Psychosexual Dysfunction.

109   The subclasses of Psychosexual Dysfunctions are: Inhibited Sexual Desire, Inhibited Sexual Excitement, Inhibited Female or Male Orgasm, Premature Ejaculation, Functional Dyspareunia, Vaginismus, or the Atypical category. All of the dysfunctions may be lifelong or acquired, developing after a period of normal functioning. They may be generalized or situational, limited to certain situations or with certain partners, and, they may be total, or partial, with varying degrees of frequency.

Inhibited Sexual Desire is a disorder consisting of persistent and pervasive inhibition of sexual desire. The judgment of inhibition is made by the clinician's taking into account factors that affect sexual desire such as age, sex, health, intensity and frequency of sexual desire, and the context of the individual's life. The category will often be used in conjunction with one or more of the other Psychosexual Dysfunction categories.

Inhibited Sexual Excitement has also been called frigidity or impotence and consists of a recurrent and persistent inhibition of sexual excitement during sexual activity, manifested by:

- in males, partial or complete failure to attain or maintain erection until completion of the sexual act.
- in females, partial or complete failure to attain or maintain the lubrication-swelling response of sexual excitement until completion of the sexual act.

Inhibited Female Orgasm consists of a recurrent and persistent inhibition of the female orgasm. It is manifested by a delay in or absence of orgasm following a normal sexual excitement phase during sexual activity that is judged by the clinician to be adequate in focus, intensity, and duration.

Inhibited Male Orgasm is a recurrent and persistent inhibition of the male orgasm as manifested by a delay in or absence of ejaculation following an adequate phase of sexual excitement.

Premature Ejaculation is characterized by ejaculation that occurs before the individual wishes it, because of recurrent and persistent absence of reasonable voluntary control of ejaculation and orgasm during sexual activity.

Functional Dyspareunia is characterized by coitus that is associated with recurrent and persistent genital pain, in either the male or the female. The disturbance is not caused exclusively by a physical disorder, and is not due to lack of lubrication, Functional Vaginismus, or another Axis I disorder.

Functional Vaginismus is the diagnosis given when there is a history of recurrent and persistent involuntary spasm of the musculature of the outer third of the vagina that interferes with coitus.

Atypical Psychosexual Dysfunction is a category that should be used for psychosexual dysfunctions that cannot be classified as a specific Psychosexual Dysfunction, such as lack of erotic sensations.

OTHER PSYCHOSEXUAL DISORDERS

110   The subclass of Other Psychosexual Disorders contains only two diagnostic entities: Ego-dystonic Homosexuality and Psychosexual Disorders Not Elsewhere Classified.

Ego-dystonic Homosexuality is only diagnosed when heterosexual arousal is persistently absent or weak and significantly interferes with initiating or maintaining wanted heterosexual relationships. In addition, there is a sustained pattern of homosexual arousal that the individual explicitly states has been unwanted and a persistent source of distress.

"Homosexuality" of DSM-II was changed to "Sexual Orientation Disturbance" in the early 70s and is now limited to this "Ego-Dystonic Homosexuality" in DSM-III.

Psychosexual Disorders Not Elsewhere Classified is a residual category whose primary manifestations are psychological disturbances related to sexuality not covered in any of the other categories in the classification of Psychosexual Disorders.

CASE VIGNETTE

A 35-year-old man has difficulty achieving and maintaining erections. Upon inquiry, he reports regular morning erections and frequent erections when fantasizing about his sexual partner. However, when he is with his sexual partner he is unable to achieve erections despite adequate or prolonged stimulation by her. He is unable to account for any undue situational circumstances which would indicate stress in his life. A physical examination showed no medical problems and he is not taking medications.

Discussion Guide

In this case there appears to be no problem in the appetitive or desire phase of sexual functioning. Stimulation is adequate for arousal and there are no medications or physical problems that would affect his ability to achieve an erection.

111   **Answer**—See Answers, Chapter 16.

Chapter 17

Factitious Disorders

GENERAL OVERVIEW

The Factitious Disorder classification is a new one for DSM-III. No similar one existed in DSM-II. DSM-III recognized the need for the inclusion of such disorders as Malingering and Factitious, and subsequently set about to define malingering and differentiate it from factitious illness.

Both Malingering and Factitious Disorders share some common features:

(1) The voluntary production of symptoms.
(2) The individual has volitional control (i.e., the timing of symptoms for maximum effect or turning the symptoms on or off).

There are distinctive features which differentiate the two:

(1) With Malingering there is an obvious, recognizable goal that will explain the symptom production.
(2) With Factitious Disorders the only motive is for the individual to assume the role of a patient.

In DSM-III, Malingering is not considered a mental disorder. Instead it is listed with Conditions Not Attributable to a Mental Disorder That Are a Focus of Attention or Treatment, and is coded on Axis I.

Webster defines "factitious" as that which is artificial or a sham. Factitious Disorders are characterized by physical or psychological symptoms that are either self-inflicted or faked by the individual as a deliberate sham and are under voluntary control. The sense of voluntary control is inferred by the observer. The inference is supported, in part, by the individual's ability to simulate illness in such a way as to avoid discovery.

The individual may inflict injury or use substances to simulate or create an illness or disorder. This behavior is considered voluntary in that it is deliberate and done with purpose, but not in the sense that the need or desire to simulate illness can be controlled. Additionally, the behavior tends to have a compulsive quality in that, even when the dangers are known, the individual seems unable to refrain from a particular behavior.

DSM-III categorizes Factitious Disorders as:

(1) With Psychological Symptoms
(2) Chronic With Physical Symptoms
(3) Atypical Factitious With Physical Symptoms

FACTITIOUS DISORDER WITH PSYCHOLOGICAL SYMPTOMS

Essential Features
This disorder has previously been referred to as Ganser Syndrome, Pseudo-psychosis and Pseudo-dementia. The symptoms produced are suggestive of a mental disorder and usually represent the individual's concept of what a mental disorder is, rather than any specific disorder.

Differential Diagnosis
Although it is very difficult to distinguish this disorder from other mental disorders, the individual with Factitious Disorder With Psychological Symptoms can sometimes be recognized by the vast array of mental symptoms that are presented. The resulting clinical picture is not characteristic of any recognizable mental disorder. For example, in a true dementia there is impairment of mental capacity and recent memory, whereas in a faked dementia there may be more loss of remote memory. Another example is the contrast between a true psychosis and a factitious one. In the faked psychosis, the observer will note that the display of symptoms are timed for maximum effect (i.e., the individual will exhibit the appropriate symptoms only when he/she feels he/she is being observed).

Diagnostic Criteria
To be given this diagnosis, the individual must meet all of the following criteria:

(1) The voluntary production of psychological symptoms.

(2) The symptoms are not explained by any other mental disorder, although they may be superimposed on one.

(3) Considering the individual's environmental circumstances, the apparent goal is to assume the role of patient.

CHRONIC FACTITIOUS DISORDER WITH PHYSICAL SYMPTOMS

Essential Features

This is the prototype for Factitious Disorders, and has also been known as Munchausen Syndrome, Hospital Hoboes, and Hospital Addiction.

Thought to be an extremely incapacitating disorder and refractory to therapy, this category should facilitate the recognition of such patients who clearly have serious psychopathology not previously classified in DSM-II. The individual with this disorder presents factitious physical symptoms so convincingly that he/she is able to obtain and sustain multiple hospitalizations. Subsequent to the multiple hospitalizations, these individuals acquire a great deal of medical information and terminology and become quite adept at fabricating physical conditions.

All organ systems are potential targets, and the symptoms presented are limited only by the individual's acquired knowledge, sophistication and imagination. Some common clinical pictures that the clinician might see include: severe right lower quadrant pain associated with nausea and vomiting, vertigo and black-out spells, back pain, and fevers of undetermined origin.

Differential Diagnosis

This disorder is most commonly confused with true medical illness and differential diagnosis is very difficult. However, there are certain elements of the individual's behavior and condition that serve as indicators to the clinician that the individual may warrant consideration for a diagnosis of Chronic Factitious Disorder With Physical Symptoms.

A clinician who notices any combination of the following behaviors or conditions should become suspicious and further investigate the individual:

- pseudologia fantastica (tellers of tall tales with great dramatic flair).
- disruptive behavior on the ward; noncompliance with hospital rules and regulations; demanding.
- extensive knowledge of hospital routines and medical terminology.
- evidence of multiple surgical intervention (i.e., "gridiron abdomen").

• fluctuating clinical course with rapid production of "complications" or new pathology once the initial workup proves to be negative.

This disorder is differentiated from other disorders such as Somatoform Disorders or Conversion Disorder by the voluntary production of the symptoms.

Diagnostic Criteria
To warrant a diagnosis of Chronic Factitious Disorder With Physical Symptoms, the following criteria must be met:

(1) The presentation of physical symptoms that are under the individual's voluntary control so convincingly that there are multiple hospitalizations.
(2) Considering the individual's environmental circumstances, the apparent goal is to assume the role of patient.

ATYPICAL FACTITIOUS DISORDER WITH PHYSICAL SYMPTOMS
This is a category for individuals who do not meet the full criteria for Chronic Factitious Disorder With Physical Symptoms. Individuals with this disorder usually present with symptoms that include self-induced conditions such as rashes or dislocation of the shoulder, but generally do not require hospitalization.

CASE VIGNETTE
A 29-year-old laboratory technician was admitted to the medical service via the emergency room for gross hematuria. The patient said that she was being treated for lupus by a physician in a different city. She also mentioned that she had Von Willebrand's Disease as a child.

On the third day of her hospitalization, a medical student mentioned to the resident that he had seen this patient several weeks prior at a different hospital in the area. A search of the patient's belongings revealed a cache of anticoagulant medication. When confronted with this information, she hurriedly signed out of the hospital against medical advice.

That evening she was admitted to another hospital in the area with similar complaints (adapted from Spitzer et al., 1981).

Discussion Guide
The Decision Tree for Differential Diagnosis of Physical Complaints and Irrational Anxiety About Physical Illness, DSM-III, pp. 346–347, may be help-

ful in reviewing this case. Key elements include: evidence of travel in the report of being treated in a different city; patient being recognized as having been seen at another hospital; the anticoagulants (which can cause hematuria); and signing out against medical advice and rapidly gaining admission elsewhere.

113   **Answer**—See Answers, Chapter 17.

Chapter 18

Disorders of Impulse Control Not Elsewhere Classified

GENERAL OVERVIEW

As the term "Not Elsewhere Classified" implies, this is a leftover category that includes disorders of impulse control that are not found in other categories, such as the Substance Use Disorders or the Paraphilias.

DSM-II contained no category that corresponds to this DSM-III classification.

This classification has six categories:

(1) Pathological Gambling
(2) Kleptomania
(3) Pyromania
(4) Intermittent Explosive Disorder
(5) Isolated Explosive Disorder
(6) Atypical Impulse Control Disorder

The diagnostic criteria for this group of disorders is characterized by three features:

(1) Experiencing tension prior to committing a harmful act.
(2) Failure to resist committing the act.
(3) Pleasure or a sense of release during the act.

In making a diagnosis it must be determined that this behavior is not due to another disorder. Further diagnostic criteria will be specified, as each disorder is individually discussed.

114

116

PATHOLOGICAL GAMBLING
This disorder is characterized by a chronic and progressive failure to resist the impulse to gamble. Subsequently, the behavior has a damaging effect on the individual's personal and professional pursuits, including loss of work due to absences to gamble, defaulting on financial responsibilities, and some criminal behavior, such as forgery, fraud, and embezzlement. It must be distinguished from social gambling or gambling behavior that is an outgrowth of a manic-like mood disturbance.

KLEPTOMANIA
Kleptomania is characterized by a recurrent failure to resist impulses to steal. Usually the objects are not taken for their monetary value or immediate use and are either given away, returned, or hidden. There is no long-term planning and no assistance from or collaboration with others. This disorder must be distinguished from ordinary stealing, Malingering, Conduct Disorder, and other such conditions.

PYROMANIA
Pyromania is characterized by a recurrent failure to resist impulses to set fires. There is an associated fascination with starting and watching fires. There may be advance preparation for setting the fire and clues may be left. The fire-setting is not motivated by monetary gain or social/political ideology.

INTERMITTENT EXPLOSIVE DISORDER
Intermittent Explosive Disorder is characterized by several discrete episodes of loss of control of aggressive impulses, resulting in assault or destruction of property. The aggressive behavior is grossly disproportionate to any precipitating psychosocial stressor. The symptoms tend to appear and remit quickly, and there is usually a report of feelings of regret. There are no signs of generalized impulsivity or aggressiveness between episodes.

This disorder must be distinguished from other disorders, such as Antisocial Personality Disorder, Dissociative Disorder, Paranoid Disorder, or Schizophrenia, Catatonic Type, and from underlying physical disorders.

ISOLATED EXPLOSIVE DISORDER
The Isolated Explosive Disorder has features similar to those of Intermittent Explosive Disorder, the primary difference being that there is a single episode

of loss of control. This single act is usually violent and externally directed, and has a disastrous impact on others. The behavior is grossly disproportionate to any precipitating psychosocial stressor. There are no indications of generalized impulsivity or aggressiveness prior to the act.

Considering the clinical information available, a diagnosis of Schizophrenia, Antisocial Personality Disorder, or other disorders is not justified; however, in some cases additional information might indicate an underlying psychosis which would preempt this diagnosis.

ATYPICAL IMPULSE CONTROL DISORDER

This is for Disorders of Impulse Control that cannot be classified anywhere else.

CASE VIGNETTE

A pregnant 27-year-old mother of six seen at the community mental health center confided that she was subject to "spells," which went away as quickly as they came. During the "spells" she struck her children and threw things at her husband with little or no provocation. She confessed that she loved her family and didn't know why she did those things. She expressed feelings of deep regret and shame and a release of tension after the incidents.

Discussion Guide

Key elements to consider include: the spells, which came and went quickly, resulting in assault; behavior that is disproportionate to any precipitating psychosocial stressor, pregnancy being the stressor; and the reports of tension and regret.

Answer—See Answers, Chapter 18.

Chapter 19

Adjustment Disorders

GENERAL OVERVIEW

The category of Adjustment Disorders is used for diagnosing disorders that are characterized by maladaptive reactions to psychosocial stressors that don't quite meet the full criteria for another specific disorder such as an Anxiety or Affective Disorder.

This category replaces the DSM-II classification of "transient situational disturbances." The DSM-II classification was applied to more or less transient disorders of any severity, including those of psychotic proportions, and was subdivided by developmental stages (i.e., "adjustment reaction" of infancy, childhood, etc.).

In DSM-III, the Adjustment Disorders classification excludes reactions of psychotic proportions such as Brief Reactive Psychosis and Schizophreniform Disorder. Adjustment Disorders are subtyped by the predominant symptoms—for example, Adjustment Disorder with Depressed Mood or Adjustment Disorder with Anxious Mood.

ESSENTIAL FEATURES

The individual with this disorder is someone who has not adapted well or has overreacted to an identifiable psychosocial stressor, resulting in the production of symptoms. Examples of such stressors include divorce, business crisis, chronic illness, interpersonal relationships, changing schools, or getting married.

The maladaptive reaction usually occurs within three months of the onset of the stressor. For example, two months after her divorce, Mary begins to express feelings of hopelessness, is frequently teary, and is depressed.

119

The maladaptive nature is evidenced by either impairment in social or occupational functioning, or the symptoms exceed the normal and expected reaction to stress. For example, Mary, who usually likes her job, now has numerous unaccustomed absences from work. However, it is surmised that the disturbance will ultimately be resolved when the stressor is terminated or when a new level of adaptation occurs. After six months, Mary is better able to accept the finality of the divorce and begins a new life as a single person.

There may be one stressor, such as divorce, or there may be more, such as business failure *and* death of a loved one. They may be recurrent, such as filing income tax returns, or continuous, such as a chronic illness. They may affect only the individual or they may affect whole groups or communities, as with an economic recession.

While the clinical syndrome is coded on Axis I, the specific stressor and severity is coded on Axis IV. For example:

> **Axis I:** Adjustment Disorder With Depressed Mood
> **Axis IV:** Psychosocial Stressors: divorce
>   Severity: Extreme—6

Differential Diagnosis
This disorder must be differentiated from some conditions, such as Other Interpersonal Problems or Phase of Life Problems.

DIAGNOSTIC CRITERIA
The following constitute criteria for Adjustment Disorders:

- a maladaptive reaction that occurs within three months of the onset of a psychosocial stressor.
- the maladaptive nature discerned by either impairment in social or occupational functioning, or symptoms exceeding the normal and expected reaction to stress.
- the disturbance is not merely a part of a pattern of overreaction to stress or an exacerbation of a mental disorder.

TYPES OF ADJUSTMENT DISORDERS
Adjustment Disorders are subclassified according to the predominant symptoms presented.

Adjustment Disorder With Depressed Mood is characterized by symptoms such as tearfulness, hopelessness, and depressed mood.

Adjustment Disorder With Anxious Mood is characterized by symptoms such as nervousness, jitteriness, and worry.

Adjustment Disorder With Mixed Emotional Features is characterized by various combinations of symptoms of depression, anxiety, and other emotions.

Adjustment Disorder With Disturbance of Conduct is characterized by behavior in which there is a violation of the rights of others or of major age-appropriate societal norms and rules.

Adjustment Disorder With Mixed Disturbance of Emotions and Conduct exhibits both emotional features and a disturbance of conduct.

Adjustment Disorder With Work (or Adademic) Inhibition exhibits inhibition in work or academic functioning in an individual whose previous performance was adequate.

Adjustment Disorder With Withdrawal is characterized by symptoms of social withdrawal without significant depressed or anxious mood.

Adjustment Disorder With Atypical Features is a category that is used when the predominant symptoms do not fall into any of the other specific categories.

CASE VIGNETTE
A 24-year-old single dental technician terminated brief psychotherapy after 10 sessions. She entered treatment two weeks after she discovered that the man she had been involved with for four months was married and wanted to stop seeing her. She reacted with bouts of crying, unaccustomed absences on three occasions from her job, and vague thoughts that the future was so pessimistic that life might not be worth the effort. She responded to mixed supportive-insight psychotherapy and toward the end of the treatment had begun dating a law student whom she met at a local cafe (adapted from Spitzer et al., 1981).

Discussion Guide
The Decision Tree for Differential Diagnosis of Mood Disturbance, DSM-III, p. 344, can be utilized in this review. There is an identifiable psychosocial stressor, finding out that the man she had been dating was married and wanted to stop seeing her. Her overreaction to the stressor produced bouts of

crying, a sense of pessimism about the future, and unaccustomed absences from work within three months. A new level of adaptation was reached and she began dating.

Answer—See Answers, Chapter 19.

Psychological Factors Affecting Physical Condition

GENERAL OVERVIEW

This is a new classification in DSM-III for the complex situations where there is a physical illness, but psychological factors are thought to be significant in initiating, exacerbating, or maintaining the condition.

In these cases, the clinician would code on Axis I, "Psychological Factors Affecting Physical Condition" to indicate the judgment that psychological factors were significant in the initiation, exacerbation, or maintenance of an Axis III condition. The physical condition is listed on Axis III.

ESSENTIAL FEATURES

The judgment that psychological factors are contributors affecting the physical condition requires some evidence of a temporal relationship between the way the individual responds to environmental stimuli, such as death of a loved one or arguments, and the initiation or exacerbation of the physical condition.

This category can be used for any physical condition where psychological factors are thought to be significant contributors. Some frequently encountered conditions include: angina, dysmenorrhea, migraine, asthma, tension headache, and low back pain.

DIAGNOSTIC CRITERIA

This diagnosis is appropriate when psychologically meaningful environmental stimuli have some temporal relationship to the initiation or exacerbation of a physical condition. The physical condition either demonstrates organic pathology or has a known pathophysiological process. It is not due to a Somatoform Disorder.

Chapter 21

Personality Disorders

GENERAL OVERVIEW

115 Personality traits are relatively stable patterns of thinking, feeling, behaving, or relating that are demonstrated over a wide range of situations. A Personality Disorder diagnosis is given when personality traits become inflexible and maladaptive, cause subjective distress, and result in significant impairment in social or occupational functioning.

There are significant differences in both the labels and the definitions of Personality Disorders from the DSM-II classification system. Previously, an attempt would be made to find the *one* Personality Disorder that would be used to identify an individual's predominant personality traits. DSM-III takes a different approach. Multiple diagnoses of Personality Disorders are appropriate if an individual meets the criteria for more than one.

Personality Disorder diagnoses can be used for children or adolescents when the traits appear to be stable early in the individual's development.

116 However, this is *unusual*. More often, some of the Personality Disorders are related to corresponding categories in the Disorders of Childhood and Adolescence if the patterns of these childhood disorders continue into adult life (i.e., after age 18). Thus a childhood Conduct Disorder could develop into an Antisocial Personality Disorder; an Oppositional Disorder into a Passive-Aggressive Personality Disorder; an Identity Disorder into Borderline Personality; Avoidant Disorder of Childhood into Avoidant Personality; and a Schizoid Disorder of Childhood or Adolescence into the Schizoid Personality Disorder.

Often Personality Disorders are accompanied by disorders of mood.

117 All Personality Disorders are coded on Axis II. A preexisting Personality Disorder can also be coded on Axis II with a psychotic disorder coded on Axis

125

I. For example: Schizophrenia, Paranoid, Chronic on Axis I and a Schizoid Personality Disorder with the word "premorbid" in parentheses on Axis II. This is to be noted if a stable personality pattern can be ascertained prior to the onset of the psychotic disorder.

Traits can also be noted on Axis II when the individual demonstrates certain traits of a particular disorder but does not meet the criteria for the full disorder. However, there is no code number for traits, and a coding of No Disorder (V71.09) or Diagnosis Deferred (799.90) should be used on Axis II if only personality traits are noted.

There are three basic clusters of Personality Disorders based on certain predominant features: "odd" or eccentric; dramatic, emotional, or erratic; and anxious or fearful.

PREDOMINANT PERSONALITY FEATURE: "ODD" OR ECCENTRIC

118   If the individual gives the impression of being "odd" or eccentric, Paranoid, Schizoid, or Schizotypal Personality Disorders should be considered.

Paranoid Personality diagnosis is used for individuals who demonstrate pervasive, unwarranted suspiciousness and mistrust of people, hypersensitivity, and restricted affective expression.

Schizoid Personality Disorder applies to individuals who demonstrate defects in the motivation and capacity to form relationships or to become emotionally involved with others, but who do not demonstrate any oddities of thinking, perceiving, or behaving. Characteristics of the Schizoid Personality are emotional coldness, indifference to the praise, criticism, or feelings of others, and very few close friendships.

Schizotypal Personality Disorder is diagnosed when there is demonstrated communication, thinking, or action that is strange or odd, but not so severely deviant to qualify for a Schizophrenia diagnosis.

Individuals with a Schizotypal diagnosis have clinical features that resemble some of the features of persons with prodromal or residual schizophrenic symptomatology. Often Schizotypal individuals were previously diagnosed as Latent, Simple, or Borderline Schizophrenia (e.g., Kety et al., 1971; Rosenthal et al., 1971). In addition to social isolation and inadequate interpersonal relationships, schizotypal personalities often demonstrate magical thinking, ideas of reference, recurrent illusions, paranoid ideation, and vague, overelaborate, or circumstantial speech without a loosening of associations.

The Schizotypal differs from the Schizoid in that no eccentricities of thought or behavior are present in the latter. Both the Schizoid and Schizotypal are newly defined categories.

PREDOMINANT PERSONALITY FEATURE: DRAMATIC, EMOTIONAL, OR ERRATIC

A second grouping of Personality Disorders focuses on individuals who present themselves in a dramatic, emotional, or erratic fashion and includes the Histrionic, Narcissistic, Antisocial, and Borderline Personality Disorders.

Histrionic Personality Disorder is characterized by overly dramatic and reactive behavior which can include emotional outbursts, craving for excitement, drawing of attention to onself, and dramatic self-presentation. Interpersonal relationships of these individuals are often shallow and they appear to be vain, egocentric, dependent, and manipulative.

The term Histrionic is used in DSM-III instead of Hysterical to remove any perjorative connotation to women and any reference to a "wandering uterus."

Borderline Personality Disorder is marked by a basic identity disturbance related to self-image, gender identity, or goals; intense interpersonal relationships; impulsive and self-damaging acts; anger dyscontrol and affective instability; problems in tolerating being alone; and chronic feelings of emptiness.

This Borderline category is more closely related to the conceptualizations of Kernberg (1967) and of Gunderson and Singer (1975) than the traditional borderline schizophrenia concept. In DSM-III the traditional concept coincides more with the Schizotypal Personality Disorder.

Narcissistic and Borderline Disorders are new diagnostic categories, even though the terms have been used in the past.

Narcissistic Personality Disorder is characterized by a grandiose sense of self-importance or uniqueness; fantasies of unlimited success or ideal love; a constant need for attention and admiration; overreaction or indifference to criticism or defeat; feelings of entitlement; exploitiveness; and lack of empathy.

Antisocial Personality Disorder is defined as a pattern of antisocial behavior which begins in adolescence (before age 15) and continues into adulthood (after age 18), during which time there is no five-year period without antisocial behavior. Antisocial Personality Disorder is now limited to individuals who display chronic violation of the rights of others in overt behavior. Individuals who in the past may have been called Antisocial Personalities because of their manipulativeness and self-aggrandizement would better be classified as Narcissistic Personalities when there is not a pattern of chronic antisocial behavior.

PREDOMINANT PERSONALITY FEATURE: ANXIOUS OR FEARFUL

120 A third grouping of Personality Disorders focuses on individuals who appear to be predominantly anxious or fearful, and includes the Avoidant, Dependent, Compulsive, and Passive-Aggressive Personality Disorders.

Avoidant Personality Disorder is a new classification which is characterized by the avoidance of desired close relationships because of a fear of rejection. This type of individual differs from the Schizoid Personality who does not desire close relationships. An Avoidant Personality would be an individual who is very sensitive to rejection, wants guarantees of uncritical acceptance, has low self-esteem, and is socially isolated, although he/she desires affection and acceptance from others.

Dependent Personality Disorder diagnosis would be given to individuals who characteristically allow others to assume responsibility for major areas of their life, lack self-confidence, and avoid having to rely on self at all costs.

Compulsive Personality Disorder omits the term obsessive to avoid confusion with the Axis I diagnosis of Obsessive Compulsive Disorder and, in actuality, has little to do with obsessions or compulsions. A compulsive individual is perfectionistic, hard-driving, and rigid, similar to the "Type A" personality identified in the stress and health behavior literature. An individual who characteristically is unduly conventional, serious, preoccupied with details and order; dedicated to work to the exclusion of others; stubbornly insists on his/her way of doing things; and is indecisive, would be classified as a Compulsive Personality Disorder.

Passive-aggressive Personality Disorder closely resembles the traditional conceptualization of passive-aggressiveness. An individual whose current and long-term functioning is marked by resisting any demands in a passive manner (e.g., procrastination, intentional inefficiency, "forgetfulness"), even when more effective and assertive behavior is possible, would be given a Passive-aggressive Personality diagnosis.

ATYPICAL, MIXED, OR OTHER PERSONALITY DISORDERS

21 There is a final general category of Personality Disorders which is used when the information available does not meet the criteria for any of the above categories but a personality diagnosis is judged appropriate.

Atypical Personality Disorder is appropriate when the clinician judges that there is a Personality Disorder but there is not enough information to make a more specific diagnosis.

Mixed Personality Disorder is used when there are features of more than one of the specific Personality Disorders, but the full criteria for any one specific Personality Disorder has not been met.

Other Personality Disorder would be used when the clinician makes the judgment that the specific Personality Disorder present is not included in the categories already mentioned. Examples of this would be Masochistic, Impulsive, or Immature Personality Disorders. There are no definitive criteria for these disorders, and such a designation relies on the knowledge and judgment of the clinician.

One code number (301.89) would be used in all three categories—Atypical, Mixed, and Other.

CASE VIGNETTE

Susan is a 26-year-old teacher's aide who came to the center for counseling. For six months she had been feeling increasingly lonely and "lost" since her sister, who is two years older, was married and moved out of town. This sister had been Susan's only real social contact; otherwise she had no girlfriends to speak of and was extremely afraid of men. Because she felt that she had very little to offer, she always anticipated that men, even if attracted, would quickly find fault with her and she would be "dropped." Although she wanted to get married, she never dated a man beyond three dates. This was her first attempt to get professional help.

Discussion Guide

There are no diagnostic decision trees relevant for all the personality disorders. However, the Decision Tree for Antisocial, Aggressive, Defiant or Oppositional Behavior, DSM-III, p. 345, does include the Antisocial Personality Disorder.

Note the social withdrawal, lack of self-esteem, and fear of social relations. The prominent features are oversensitivity and the desire for social relations.

122   **Answer**—See Answers, Chapter 21.

Chapter 22

Specific Developmental Disorders

GENERAL OVERVIEW

Specific Developmental Disorders are disorders of circumscribed areas of development or learning which are not due to another disorder.

To make a diagnosis of a Specific Developmental Disorder, it is necessary to first rule out Mental Retardation, physical or organic impairment, and Pervasive Developmental Disorders. Developmental lags that are due to these other disorders are not diagnosed as Specific Developmental Disorders. For example, a blind child will be unable to read but should not be diagnosed as having a Developmental Reading Disorder.

Developmental Disorders are related to biological maturation and expected functioning levels for normal children. However, a biological dysfunction is not assumed to be the cause of the disorder.

The disorders in this class are subclassified according to the predominant area of functioning affected and include Developmental Reading, Arithmetic, Language, and Mixed and Atypical Specific Developmental Disorders. These diagnoses are not to be used to describe a "slow learner." There should be a significant discrepancy between actual and expected levels of performance for a diagnosis to be made. Determining what constitutes a significant delay demands clinical judgment and knowledge of normal development. The guideline of at least a one- or two-year delay is used in DSM-III for disorders which appear in school years.

These diagnoses are used primarily for children and are found in the section on Disorders Usually First Evident in Infancy, Childhood, or Adolescence. However, they should also be used for adults who still show clinically significant signs of the disorder.

124　　Specific Developmental Disorders, coded on Axis II, often occur in conjunction with other disorders which would be noted on Axis I. For example, Conduct Disorder or Attention Deficit Disorder with Hyperactivity.

In DSM-II these diagnoses were all classified under the heading "specific learning disturbance."

DEVELOPMENTAL READING DISORDER

125　The keynote of the Developmental Reading Disorder is a significant impairment in the development of reading skills. In order to make this diagnosis a standardized, individually administered I.Q. test is needed to establish intellectual capacity. Reading skills tests and school performance should indicate functioning below expected level for education, chronological and mental age. This disorder has been previously referred to as "dyslexia."

DEVELOPMENTAL ARITHMETIC DISORDER

The keynote of this disorder is a significant impairment in the development of arithmetic skills. The diagnostic criteria are the same as those for a Reading Disorder, but focused on arithmetic.

DEVELOPMENTAL LANGUAGE DISORDER

126　The Developmental Language Disorder is subdivided into two types: a Receptive Type, when the problem lies in the comprehension of oral language, and an Expressive Type, when the problem is in expressing verbal language. These are not the same as "aphasia," which is a loss of language already acquired.

In the Expressive Type of Language Disorder there are indications that the individual does have inner language and can understand basic concepts but is unable to verbally express them. In the Receptive Type there exists both the inability to understand language or develop inner language and the inability to express concepts in verbal language.

DEVELOPMENTAL ARTICULATION DISORDER

127　The basic feature of the Developmental Articulation Disorder is the consistent misarticulation of the later-acquired speech sounds not due to another disorder or physical impairment. The types of sounds typically found in this disorder are sh, r, th, f, z, l, or ch.

MIXED SPECIFIC DEVELOPMENTAL DISORDER

The diagnosis of Mixed Specific Developmental Disorder is used when there is more than one Developmental Disorder of the same degree of impairment. If there are different degrees of impairment, multiple diagnoses of the specific Developmental Disorders should be made.

ATYPICAL SPECIFIC DEVELOPMENTAL DISORDER

The diagnosis of Atypical Specific Developmental Disorder is used when there is a specific developmental delay that cannot be placed in any of the other categories.

CASE VIGNETTE

George is a fourth grader who is having difficulty in school. He gets along well with other children but has poor academic performance. George is flunking reading and spelling and having difficulty in science. He is passing math, art, and physical education. On the Wechsler Intelligence Scale for Children, he obtained a full scale I.Q. score of 100 with a verbal score of 95 and a performance score of 103. On an individual achievement test, George's reading comprehension score was at grade level 1.6, his spelling score was at grade level 2.0, and his math score was at grade level 3.2. There were no notable problems at home with the exception of the parents' difficulty in getting George to do his homework.

Discussion Guide

This case can be reviewed using the Decision Tree for Differential Diagnosis of Academic or Learning Difficulties, DSM-III, p. 348.

This individual is having school difficulties in areas which depend on reading for adaptive functioning. He is performing two years below expected grade level although he has normal intelligence. Arithmetic skills are basically intact and only mildly affected by the Reading Disorder; minor problems in arithmetic are probably due to difficulty with mathematical word problems.

128 **Answer**—See Answers, Chapter 22.

Section IV

Application

Chapter 23

Coding Procedures

GENERAL OVERVIEW

As the name implies, DSM-III is designed for recording diagnostic *and* statistical information on individuals seen in a psychiatric setting. In order to be able to retrieve valuable information on individuals treated, and meet the goals of DSM-III, the diagnosis given must accurately reflect the individual's condition. The clinician must include the *specific* information needed to adequately code the diagnosis. This chapter will highlight technical aspects of coding DSM-III disorders and outline some additional capacities of the system.

AXIS I AND AXIS II CODES

On pp. 15–19 of DSM-III there is a listing of all the code numbers and terms that would appear on Axis I or Axis II. Axis II codes and categories are indicated with boldface boxes around the disorders that could appear on this axis (Specific Developmental Disorders, Personality Disorders, and Additional Codes). All the codes and categories which are not enclosed in the boxes are to be used exclusively on Axis I in the DSM-III system.

Additional Codes

129 There is a section of all Additional Codes which represent general diagnostic statements. These statements have been discussed in the section on levels of diagnostic certainty in Chapter 3 and will be reviewed here.

If, after an examination of the individual, the clinician determines that there is no mental disorder present on Axis I and/or Axis II, the term *No Diagnosis* is used with the code V71.09.

When there is insufficient information available to make a diagnostic judgment on Axis I and/or Axis II, the term *Diagnosis Deferred* with the code 799.90 is used.

When enough information is available to rule out a psychotic disorder, but further specification is not possible, the term *Unspecified Mental Disorder (nonpsychotic)* with the code 300.90 is noted on Axis I.

If enough information is available to determine the presence of a psychotic disorder, but further specification is not possible, the term *Atypical Psychosis* with the code 298.90 from the section on Psychotic Disorders Not Elsewhere Classified would be noted on Axis I.

Fifth Digit Codes

130   There are six diagnostic classes in DSM-III which use the fifth digit of the code to indicate the course, severity, or associated features of a particular disorder. It is important to remember to include this information in making a diagnosis from one of these classes. Otherwise, the diagnosis will be incomplete and cannot be properly coded. Whenever an "X" appears in the fifth digit, additional information is needed.

The categories which use a fifth digit subtype or other qualifying term are: Disorders Usually First Evident in Infancy, Childhood, or Adolescence; Organic Mental Disorders; Substance Use Disorders; Schizophrenic Disorders; Affective Disorders; and Psychosexual Disorders. Examples of each of the categories using a fifth digit subtype follow.

131   **Mental Retardation.** In order to make a complete diagnosis of Mental Retardation, the presence or absence of behavioral symptoms that require attention or treatment must be noted. The fifth digit code is "1" if there are other behavioral symptoms requiring attention or treatment and that are not part of another disorder. The fifth digit code is "0" if there are no other behavioral symptoms.

132   Severe Mental Retardation, code 318.1(x) is not a complete diagnosis. A complete diagnosis would be Severe Mental Retardation, Without Other Behavioral Symptoms, code 318.10.

Pervasive Developmental Disorders. In the diagnosis of Pervasive Developmental Disorders, the designation of the presence of a full syndrome or a residual state must be noted. If a full syndrome is present, the fifth digit code is "0." The fifth digit code for a residual state is "1."

For example, the diagnosis of Infantile Autism, 299.0(x) is not complete unless the clinician notes whether there is a full syndrome present (299.01), or it is in a residual state (299.00).

Organic Mental Disorders. When a diagnosis from the subclass of Dementias arising in the Senium or Presenium is made, the associated features must be coded to make the diagnosis complete. Fifth digit codes are: 1—with delirium; 2—with delusions; 3—with depression; and 0—uncomplicated.

For example, Multi-infarct Dementia, code 290.4(x) is coded to the fifth digit, 290.42 for Multi-infarct Dementia, With Delusions.

For Dementia associated with alcohol, the severity of the Dementia must also be noted for a complete diagnosis in the subclass of the Organic Mental Disorders. Fifth digit codes for severity are: 1—mild; 2—moderate; 3—severe; and 0—unspecified.

So the diagnostic code for Dementia Associated With Alcoholism, 291.2(x) is not complete without the coded severity; for example, Dementia Associated With Alcohol, Mild is coded 291.21.

133   **Substance Use Disorder.** Diagnosing a Substance Use Disorder requires that the clinician code in the fifth digit the pattern of use. Fifth digit codes are: 1—continuous; 2—episodic; 3—in remission; and 0—unspecified.

134   For example, Opioid Abuse, code 305.5(x) is coded to the fifth digit, 305.51, for Opioid Abuse, Continuous.

Schizophrenic Disorders. Fifth digit codes for Schizophrenic Disorders are: 1—subchronic; 2—chronic; 3—subchronic with acute exacerbation; 4—chronic with acute exacerbation; 5—in remission; and 0—unspecified.

Schizophrenia, Paranoid, code 295.3(x) is coded to the fifth digit, for example, to notate a chronic condition, 295.32.

135   **Affective Disorders.** Diagnosing a major depressive episode requires some indication of whether the depression is in remission or is accompanied by psychotic features or melancholia. Fifth digit codes are: 6—in remission; 4—with psychotic features (here the unofficial non-ICD-9-CM fifth digit 7 may be used instead to indicate that the psychotic features are mood-incongruent); 3—with melancholia; 2—without melancholia; and 0—unspecified.

136   To code the diagnosis of Major Depression, Recurrent, the code 296.3(x) must be taken to the fifth digit to indicate, for example, in remission. The code would be 296.36.

Similarly, in the diagnosis of a manic episode it is necessary for the clinician to note whether the condition is: in remission, fifth digit code 6; with or without psychotic features, fifth digit code 4 or 2; or unspecified, code 0. Bipolar Disorder, Manic, for example, is coded 296.4(x). Psychotic features are noted as 296.44, Bipolar Disorder, Manic With Psychotic Features.

Psychosexual Disorders. The final diagnostic category which uses the fifth digit coding for greater specificity is the Psychosexual Disorders. In the diagnosis of a Gender Identity Disorder, the sexual history of the individual is coded in the fifth digit as: 1—asexual; 2—homosexual; 3—heterosexual; or 0—unspecified.

For example, the diagnosis of Transsexualism, code 302.5(x), is incomplete without a notation of sexual history. If there is a history of homosexuality, then the complete code would be 302.52.

V CODES

137   The section on Conditions Not Attributable to a Mental Disorder That Are a Focus of Attention or Treatment has included a brief list adapted from ICD-9-CM of factors that would bring an individual into contact with mental health services. The description of these "V Code" conditions is in DSM-III, pp. 331–334.

It is important to remember that all V Codes, with the exception of V71.09—No Diagnosis, are placed on Axis I. V71.09 may be used with either Axis I or Axis II. The DSM-III list of V Codes is only a selection of the ICD-9-CM list of V Codes. Certain agencies or clinicians may be interested in tracking other conditions, like Alcoholism in the Family, or Illegitimate Pregnancy, which are not included in the DSM-III list but do appear in ICD-9-CM.

AXIS III CODES

138   Physical conditions that are relevant for the understanding or management of an individual are noted on Axis III. The codes for these conditions are found in ICD-9 and are not included in DSM-III. Ordinarily, the clinician will simply write down the condition and leave the coding to a medical records person or department.

Different types of information can be included on Axis III that may be of interest to a facility or clinician. In addition to diseases, a section of ICD-9 called E Codes allows for the notation of suicide and the means used for a suicide attempt, child battering by various persons, and other physical conditions caused by accidents or adverse affects of certain treatment.

AXIS IV

139   When noting the level of psychosocial stressors on Axis IV, the rating (coded 1-7) and term (None—Catastrophic) should be used. If no information is available on psychosocial stressors, then a code of "0" for Unspecified is used. In addition to noting the code and term, the clinician should also list the stressors.

AXIS V CODES

When indicating the highest level of adaptive functioning on Axis V, both the rating (coded 1-7) and the term (Superior—Grossly Impaired) should be used. If no information is available, then a code of "0" for Unspecified is used.

Chapter 24

Case Vignettes

GENERAL OVERVIEW

Five vignettes have been developed to provide short, comprehensive, clinical pictures for practice in diagnosing with the DSM-III classification system. Although the five vignettes are based on actual cases, details have been summarized and changed to protect the confidentiality of the clients/patients. Each vignette includes the basic information needed to make a multiaxial diagnosis.

In a format similar to the one in Table 13, write diagnoses and the appropriate codes for Axes I and II. Place the principal diagnosis on Axis I, number one. If the principal diagnosis is an Axis II diagnosis, write (Principal Diagnosis) following the name of the disorder. Note relevant physical conditions on Axis III.

The multiaxial evaluations of the five cases represent the consensus of five clinicians from the Texas Research Institute of Mental Sciences who helped develop the material. The answers provided (included in the Answer Section) are not meant to represent the only possible diagnoses of these cases. The discussion guide following each case provides information about possible alternate diagnoses depending on the clinical evaluation of the very brief vignettes.

CASE #1—SARAH

Summary

Sarah is a 36-year-old housewife and mother doing some part-time work as a bookkeeper. She is referred by her gynecologist, who had prescribed a sedative for her disturbed sleep, but found that her problems were more complex and extensive.

TABLE 13
Diagnostic Appraisal

AXIS I: Psychiatric Syndromes   **CODES**
  1. _____   ___ ___ ___.___ ___
  2. _____   ___ ___ ___.___ ___
  3. _____   ___ ___ ___.___ ___

AXIS II: Personality and Specific Developmental Disorders
  1. _____   ___ ___ ___.___ ___
  2. _____   ___ ___ ___.___ ___
  3. _____   ___ ___ ___.___ ___

AXIS III: Physical Disorders

  _____   ___ ___ ___.___ ___

  _____   ___ ___ ___.___ ___

AXIS IV: Psychosocial Stressors (check one)
  (1)   (2)   (3)   (4)   (5)   (6)   (7)
  None Minimal Mild Moderate Severe Extreme Catastrophic

List stressors _____

_____

_____

AXIS V: Highest Level of Adaptive Functioning Past Year (check one)
  (1)   (2)   (3) (4) (5)   (6)   (7)
  Superior Very Good Good Fair Poor Very Poor Grossly Impaired

Prior to the onset of the current symptoms, she was content, energetic, involved in a part-time college course and enjoying what seemed to be the best phase in her life. She had plenty of energy for her housework, gourmet cooking, occasional bridge with friends, and managing a household with three children.

Four months ago, her husband was promoted to a job requiring that he travel three or four days a week. This left her with sole responsibility for the entire household. This situation was aggravated by her older son's becoming moody, obstinate, and difficult to manage. Characteristically, Sarah was reluctant to burden her husband with these matters.

For about the last three months, nothing seems the way it used to be. She is sad all the time, afraid that she won't be able to manage all her responsibilities, afraid of failing. She dropped her college work because she couldn't concentrate; lately, she has missed work because of feeling too tired.

She has lost her interest in cooking, which only seems like a chore. Food is unappealing to her; sometimes she can hardly swallow it. She has lost 12 pounds in the last two months. She would not consider suicide, but is so despondent that she wishes she could be dead.

She went to the gynecologist for a complete checkup. No physical problems were found, but the doctor prescribed a sedative for her disturbed sleep. When she called to refill the prescription last week, she indicated that she was really no better and that she could hardly get moving in the mornings. The gynecologist then referred her for this evaluation.

Sarah appears haggard; she is tearful, dabbing at her eyes with a tissue which she wrings in her hands. She sounds weary and exhausted. She seems bewildered by her inability to throw off this mood and feel normal again. She describes a pervasive inability to enjoy anything anymore.

Multiaxial Diagnosis—See Answers, Chapter 24, a.

Discussion

   Axis I. This case illustrates a primary disorder of mood, with development of a full depressive syndrome over the last three months (after the husband's promotion). Since this is a full blown syndrome, AdjustmentDisorder with Depressed Mood is ruled out. She never had a manic episode, so this is in the Unipolar Depressive Group. Sarah meets the quota for symptoms of Major Depression. Dysthymic Disorder is ruled out by the brevity of her symptoms and their severity. There are enough "endogenous" features—weight loss, disturbed sleep, distinct despondent quality to mood—to set the severity level at "with melancholia." This is clearly her first episode.

   Axis II. Sarah was an enthusiastic and vigorous person before the onset of the disorder, with no evidence of maladaptive character traits. Many industrious patients are labeled as "compulsive" without real inspection to see if the distinct qualities of compulsive traits are present (rigid, aloof, demanding, ruinously perfectionistic). Deferring diagnosis on Axis II is acceptable if one feels a need for more personality information.

   Axis III. Examination by her physician ruled out physical problems.

   Axis IV. The role of two psychosocial stressors is clear: the husband's absences and the son's troublesome behavior. Other difficulties are faced, but only these two stressors are clearly involved in initiating and exacerbating her symptoms. Thus, the rating is Moderate—4.

Axis V. The demands and complexity of her many roles are considerable, but not quite as much as the toughest roles encountered. Thus, the consensus is that her Highest Level of Adaptive Functioning during the past calendar year is Very Good—2.

CASE #2—RACHAEL

Summary
Rachael is a 26-year-old, Jewish female from an upper-middle-class family who has completed a bachelor's degree in sociology. She has one older sister, Lauren, whom she idealizes and of whom she is extremely jealous. Rachael has a considerable amount of anger and ambivalence toward her parents by whom she feels ignored.

Rachael is very intelligent and verbal. She talks openly of her problems with mildly pressured speech and some agitation. Her dress and grooming are attractive. She is oriented to time, place, and person, and her mood is a mixture of anxiety and depression. While discussing her impending divorce, her eyes fill with tears.

She begins the interview worried that what she says will not be understood and is slightly suspicious that what she says will not be confidential.

Approximately two years ago Rachael married a clinical psychology graduate student. They separated about six weeks ago after her husband learned from his brother about Rachael's infidelities. He became furious and filed for divorce. Since that time she has become more anxious and depressed. Rachael has moved into an apartment and feels lonely and isolated. She is afraid to meet friends who know her husband for fear he has told them about her, and she is reluctant to make new friends. Although she continues to work as a legal secretary for the firm she has been with for the past year and one-half, her efficiency and productivity have fallen below her usual, competent standards. Additionally, she is having difficulties with fellow employees and has gone to bed with some of the lawyers of the firm.

Reluctantly, Rachael admits that she has had difficulty controlling her behavior for a long time. She has had episodes of excessive drinking and drug usage, has engaged in impulsive shoplifting of clothes and promiscuous heterosexual and homosexual behavior. She is extremely angry at the men she has been intimate with and feels dirty and used.

Since her youth, Rachael has been an obsessional person and has never felt very secure. She has made several suicidal gestures in the past in order to "let off steam," but is not currently suicidal.

Multiaxial Diagnosis—See Answers, Chapter 24, b.

Discussion
Axis I. The diagnosis of Adjustment Disorder with Mixed Emotional Features assumes that the depression, dysphoria, and anger presented are largely a reaction to the separation from her husband and the pending divorce. This diagnosis assumes that the current level of depression and anger are not explained by the Borderline Diagnosis. If a clinician judged that the current depression was simply an exacerbation of the Borderline Personality Disorder, then no diagnosis would be made on Axis I. A number of individuals presented with this case have used a diagnosis of Dysthymic Disorder on Axis I. However, the depression, even if present prior to the separation, seems to have been managed by acting-out behavior rather than depressive symptomatology. Thus, a Dysthymic diagnosis does not seem appropriate.

Axis II. The patient clearly meets the criteria of the Borderline Personality Disorder. Although the patient comes in complaining of depression, her Borderline Personality appears to be the central problem in her life and, hence, the principal diagnosis. The fact that an Axis II diagnosis is considered the principal diagnosis must be noted on Axis II. Since so many of the acting-out behaviors, such as drug usage and shoplifting, are part of a Borderline Personality Disorder, these behaviors do not merit additional diagnoses on Axis I.

Axis III. There are no current relevant physical conditions.

Axis IV. Since the marital separation and many changes in her life contributed to either the diagnosis of Adjustment Disorder or the exacerbation of the Borderline Disorder, they should be noted on Axis IV and coded as Severe —5. If psychosocial stressors were judged to play little or no part in this individual's disorders, then a much lower rating of stress could be used.

Avis V. Although the patient leads a chaotic life, she has been able, for the most part, to maintain a job and function well on the job during the past year. Social relations are impaired and have been over the past year in spite of the patient's being married. A rating of Fair—4, as the Highest Level of Adaptive Functioning over the past year, reflects both her ability to function and her problems with social relations. Her current level of adaptive functioning would be worse, but Axis V necessitates an assessment of functioning over the past year, not the past two months. Again, some spread in rating the highest level on Axis V was experienced in previous training sessions.

CASE #3—MARK

Summary

Mark is a 10-year-old boy who was referred by Child Welfare authorities.

Background information reveals that pregnancy and birth were uncomplicated. Developmental milestones are within normal limits. He has experienced the usual childhood illnesses, but has had no serious physical illness. A sister, four years older, is Mark's only sibling in his intact middle-class family. He has had playmates in the neighborhood and has participated in socialization experiences through his extended family and church.

During the interview, Mark is unresponsive and moves somewhat aimlessly around the room. He makes sounds but no identifiable speech. When presented with toys, he seems disinterested in them and does not engage in cooperative play. At times, he sits in his chair staring off in the distance and waving his hands in the air. However, he finds it difficult to sit still, moves about the room a great deal, and has to be restrained by the interviewer.

When Mark was five years old, his father was burned in an accident at a chemical plant. The father was hospitalized for several weeks, and eventually died from these injuries. When visiting his father, the child would often scream and pull at the bandages covering his father's burns. It was at this point that Mark's mother began to notice "a change" in him.

After his father's death, Mark began exhibiting perseverative speech. For no identifiable reason, he began having "outbursts" of crying and excitability during which he could not be comforted. At times, he would laugh or smile to himself. His mother reported that Mark stopped playing with his toys and would become preoccupied "waving his hands" or "moving his fingers." He began to exhibit head-banging, especially when a change was made in his routine.

Currently, Mark has no language. He continues to have unexplained "temper outbursts" with self-mutilative behavior. He requires careful supervision as he lacks appropriate fear reactions and has also experienced a regression in self-help skills. A pediatric examination revealed no medical problems. Child Welfare authorities are investigating proper placement facilities as his mother reports she can no longer care for the child.

Multiaxial Diagnosis—See Answers, Chapter 24, c.

Discussion
    Axis I. The principal diagnosis in this case is Childhood Onset Pervasive Development Disorder, Full Syndrome. In this child there is a gross and sustained impairment in many areas of functioning, especially social relationships, which began after age five. He continues to demonstrate the presence of the full syndrome up to the present time. The age of onset distinguishes this disorder from Infantile Autism. If delusions, hallucinations, or marked loosening of associations could be identified, then a diagnosis of Schizophrenia would need to be considered.
    Although this child is at present untestable, an additional diagnosis of Mental Retardation would also be given to note the presence of significantly subaverage intellectual functioning and impairment in adaptive functioning.

    Axis II. No diagnosis would be appropriate on Axis II since the specific areas of developmental delay are all accounted for by the pervasive Developmental Disorder diagnosis and would not merit a diagnosis on Axis II.

    Axis III. A pediatric exam yielded no relevant physical conditions.

    Axis IV. Even though the father's traumatic death occurred five years prior to the present assessment, this event was critical in the onset of the disorder and is mentioned on Axis IV. A coding of Extreme—6 seems most appropriate. If the father's death was judged to be a catastrophic event, a rating of 7 could be used. In general, some spread in the rating of Axis IV would be experienced in doing this exercise.

    Axis V. Since Mark has functioned at the level demonstrated in the interview during the entire preceding year, a rating of Grossly Impaired—7 was judged to be most appropriate.

CASE #4—JACK

Summary
Jack is a 25-year-old geology graduate student brought for treatment by his father, who is a minister. Jack dropped out of school three months ago and returned home. Rather than recovering his ability to pursue his studies, he became more withdrawn and self-absorbed, convinced that he had been chosen for a special religious mission.

The interview is chaotic. Jack is suspicious and distrustful. There is a helter-skelter, unpredictable quality to his behavior and responses. Occasionally, he abruptly stops speaking and makes a peculiar gesture by crossing his fingers over his forehead. Some of the time he responds to questions, but at other times he is prompted by some fleeting internal preoccupation. He shifts from concern about his studies to religiosity, to sexual conflicts, to his problematic relationship with his father.

Jack believes that an Indian medicine man is using voodoo on him to brainwash him into desiring oral sex. He hears the voice of the medicine man and the voice of God. Sometimes, the two voices argue over him. His hand gesture is a sign of the cross designed to ward off the medicine man's evil spell.

Jack came from a very conventional and moralistic household. He was rather inexperienced when he undertook his studies for his doctorate in Canada a year and a half ago. Jack has been unable to reconcile his moralistic upbringing with the realities of adult heterosexual life. He fell in love with Jennie, a free-spirited classmate, who challenged his traditional views. She felt they should live together and establish sexual compatibility. Jack was balky and hesitant. Jennie became impatient and broke off with him a year ago.

Jack had been a bright and promising student, but his independent graduate research plans were too sweeping and impractical. He would not heed his advisors' suggestions and launched into the effort eight or nine months ago. It was while alone in the woods that he began to hear the voice of the medicine man. He began to feel that his advisors were against him, that his mission was to be tested by God. He couldn't pursue his schoolwork, as the "mission" consumed his attention. Since arriving at home, he has become convinced that the medicine man is disguising himself as other people all around. The voices, which were intermittent at first, are nearly constant now.

Jack has been in excellent physical health and has never consumed drugs.

Multiaxial Diagnosis—See Answers, Chapter 24, d.

Discussion

Axis I. There is a marked drop in the level of functioning and a wide array of disturbed mental functioning. This is not a picture that is the outgrowth of organicity or mood disturbance. The major features are the bizarre delusions, hallucinations, bizarre gestures, and religiosity. Criterion A for Schizophrenia (Paranoid Disorder is ruled out) is clearly met. The differentiation along paranoid lines establishes that the type of Schizophrenia is Paranoid. The prodromal symptoms were evident around a year ago, and the active psychotic symptoms have been continuous for eight or nine months. Jack is still in the psychotic phase, so the course is designated "subchronic." This is not "subchronic with acute exacerbation" because the psychotic symptoms never did subside and reemerge.

Axis II. There may have been a long-standing personality problem present, but the chaotic state of the interview does not allow enough clear information to be gathered about Axis II. "Diagnosis Deferred" is the best approach to Axis II.

Axis III. Jack stated "a perfect record" concerning physical problems, so 'None Known" is the Axis III selection.

Axis IV. The vignette pinpoints two psychosocial stressors involved in triggering the disorder: jilting by the girlfriend a year ago and the taking on of an unstructured research task. Other elements are present, but they have to do with his personal vulnerability demonstrated by his inability to reconcile values. The rating for Axis IV is Moderate—4.

Axiv V. Over the past calendar year, there has not been a sustained period when Jack was doing well. He was embroiled in his troubles over Jennie a year ago, and, even though he was enrolled in graduate school, he was not on good terms with his advisors. The consensus for Axis V is Poor—5.

CASE #5—GERALD

Summary
Gerald is a 56-year-old engineer who has been involuntarily retired for four months. He is accompanied to the interview and assisted through it by his wife, who is attentive, protective, and concerned.

Gerald has been with the same engineering firm for 19 years. He has established a reputation as "the human computer" because of his aloof, "all business" manner, his encyclopedic knowledge, and his machine-like dedication to his work. He was functioning in his accustomed fashion until a gradual change set in two or three years ago. Without any source of external stress, there was a progressive decline in his work, in his ability to make decisions, and then, in his memory.

A year and half ago, he was removed from his role as division head and given a lateral promotion (a euphemism for being "farmed out" to less demanding duties). He was unable to get the hang of his new role and his forgetfulness eventually rendered him unable to continue at work at all. Four months ago, he was terminated. At home, his condition has continued the slow decline. He has alarmed his wife by forgetting to lock the doors, forgetting to turn off the water, forgetting to turn off the burner on the stove. He became confused while driving, got lost on the freeway, and now his wife does all the driving.

Gerald hasn't wanted to see a doctor; he tries to minimize or explain away his failing mental powers. He claims to be the same as ever, but family friends confirm a personality change that his wife has noticed. He was never a warm person, but he has become cranky, irritable, and suspicious of people's motives. Careful questioning reveals no frank delusion formation.

In the interview, Gerald is somewhat disheveled and bewildered, but is defensive about his defects. He can't recall his correct age, even after a reminder. He is disoriented and has uncertain recall of recent events, but intact recall of the distant past. He performs dismally on attempts at calculation, excusing his poor performance as based on his usual reliance on a calculator (which he at first calls a calendar).

Aside from gout, Gerald has no known medical disorder. There is a suggestion that his own father may have developed a similar mental disorder in his 50s.

Multiaxial Diagnosis—See Answers, Chapter 24, e.

Discussion

Axis I. This case illustrates the syndrome of Dementia. The amnestic features are joined by personality change and difficulties with computation. A degree of depression, though not really evident in the interview, is superimposed. While he has become cranky and suspicious, he has definitely not developed delusions. The hint of a family history is strongly suggestive of Primary Degenerative Dementia, as is the stable gradual decline. There is no history of little strokes.

Axis II. Gerald's usual premorbid personality is no longer evident, but there is enough information to establish that he displayed marked compulsive traits and probably a Compulsive Personality Disorder before the onset of the Dementia, which has altered and obscured his previous personality features.

Axis III. There is no known physical condition for Axis III other than gout, which is unrelated to the Axis I disorder.

Axis IV. The matter of psychosocial stressors is complicated in this case. This disorder came on slowly out of nowhere and has progressed to incapacitation. There clearly were no psychosocial stressors involved in precipitating the disorder. A number of setbacks have occurred as consequences of the Dementia (loss of job, loss of status, loss of friends), but none of these has exacerbated any of the features of the Dementia. It is important to recognize that while stress points may be found, Axis IV is confined to listing *those psychosocial stressors which initiate or exacerbate the Axis I disorder.*

Axis V. Gerald, according to his wife's report, was really nonfunctional even though employed during the past year. For this reason, the consensus for Axis V was Very Poor—6.

Appendix: Answers

Chapter 2
Sherlock Holmes

Chapter 7
  a. Axis IV: Psychosocial stressors: death of a grandparent; change in neighborhood and residence.
     Severity: Severe—5
  b. Axis IV: Psychosocial stressors: new boss with change in style of supervision.
     Severity: Mild—3

Chapter 8
  a. Axis V: Fair—4
  b. Axis V: Good—3

Chapter 9
  a. Axis I: Childhood Onset Pervasive Developmental Disorder 299.9(x)
  b. Axis I: Conduct Disorder, Socialized, Nonaggressive 312.21

Chapter 10
  a. Axis I: Valium Dependence, Continuous 304.11
  b. Axis I: Alcohol Withdrawal Delirium 291.00

Chapter 11
  a. Axis I: Schizophrenia, Disorganized, Subchronic 295.11

b. Axis I: Brief Reactive Psychosis 298.80
c. Axis I: Paranoia 297.10

Chapter 12
Axis I: Bipolar Disorder, Manic, with Mood-Congruent Psychotic Features 296.44

Chapter 13
Axis I: Panic Disorder 300.01

Chapter 14
Axis I: Hypochondriasis 300.70

Chapter 15
Axis I: Psychogenic Fugue 300.13

Chapter 16
Axis I: Inhibited Sexual Excitement 302.72

Chapter 17
Axis I: Chronic Factitious Disorder with Physical Symptoms 301.51

Chapter 18
Axis I: Intermittent Explosive Disorder 312.34

Chapter 19
Axis I: Adjustment Disorder with Depressed Mood 309.00

Chapter 21
Axis II: Avoidant Personality Disorder 301.82

Chapter 22
Axis II: Developmental Reading Disorder 315.00

Chapter 24
a. **Multiaxial Diagnosis**
Axis I: Major Depression, Single Episode with Melancholia 296.23
Axis II: No Diagnosis   V71.09
          or Diagnosis Deferred   799.90
Axis III: None Known

Axis IV: Moderate—4
Husband's absence, turmoil with son
Axis V: Very Good—2

b. Multiaxial Diagnosis

Axis I:	Adjustment Disorder with Mixed Emotional Features	309.28
	or Adjustment Disorder with depressed mood	309.00
	or No Diagnosis	V71.09
Axis II:	Borderline Personality Disorder (Principal Diagnosis)	301.83
Axis III:	None	

Axis IV: Severe—5
Separation, loss of friends, and difficulties with fellow workers, change of residence.
Axis V: Fair—4

c. Multiaxial Diagnosis

Axis I:	Childhood Onset Pervasive Developmental Disorder, Full Syndrome	299.90
	Mental Retardation, Unspecified	319.01
Axis II:	No Diagnosis	V71.09
Axis III:	None	

Axis IV: Extreme—6
Father's accidental and traumatic death
Axis V: Grossly Impaired—7

d. Multiaxial Diagnosis

Axis I:	Schizophrenia, Paranoid, Subchronic	295.31
Axis II:	Diagnosis Deferred	799.90
Axis III:	None Known	

Axis IV: Moderate—4
Jilted by girlfriend, unstructured research task
Axis V: Poor—5

e. Multiaxial Diagnosis

Axis I:	Primary Degenerative Dementia, Presenile Onset, with Depression	290.13
	or, Uncomplicated	290.10
Axis II:	Compulsive Personality Disorder (premorbid)	301.40

or Compulsive Personality traits   V71.09

Axis III: Gout
Axis IV: None—1
Axis V: Very Poor—6

References

Preface

    Webb, L. J., Gold, R. S., Johnstone, E. E., & DiClemente, C. C.: Accuracy of DSM-III diagnosis following a training program. *Am. J. Psychiatry*, 138: 376–378, 1981.

Chapter 2

    Spitzer, R. L., Skodol, A. E., Gibbon, M., & Williams, J. B. W.: "DSM-III: Psychiatric Diagnosis for the 1980's." December 6–8, 1979, New York City.

Chapter 7

    Holmes, T. H., & Rahe, R. H.: The social readjustment rating scale. *J. Psychosomatic Research*, 11: 213–218, 1967.

Chapter 8

    Newman, F. L., & Rinkus, A. J.: Level of functioning, clinical judgment, and mental health service evaluation. *Evaluation and the Health Professions*, 1: 175–194, 1978.

Chapter 13

    Marks, I.: *Fear and Phobias*. New York: Academic Press, 1968.
    Klein, D. F., Zitrin, C. M., & Woerner, M. G.: Antidepressants, anxiety, panic and phobia. In: *Psychopharmacology: A Generation of Progress*. Edited by Lipton, M. A., DiMascio, A., & Killan, K. F. New York: Raven Press, 1978.
    Zitrin, C. M., Klein, D. F., & Woerner, M. G.: Behavior therapy, sup-

portive psychotherapy, imipramine and phobias. *Archives of General Psychiatry*, 35: 307–316, 1978.

Chapter 16

Masters, W. H., & Johnson, V. E.: *Human Sexual Inadequacy*. Boston: Little, Brown, 1970.

Kaplan, H. S.: *Disorders of Sexual Desire*. New York: Brunner/Mazel, 1979.

Kaplan, H. S.: *The New Sex Therapy*. New York: Brunner/Mazel, 1974.

Chapter 17

Spitzer, R. L., Skodol, A. E., Gibbon, M., & Williams, J. B. W.: *DSM-III Case Book*. Washington, D.C.: American Psychiatric Association, 1981.

Chapter 19

Spitzer, R. L., Skodol, A. E., Gibbon, M., & Williams, J. B. W.: *DSM-III Case Book*. Washington, D.C.: American Psychiatric Association, 1981.

Chapter 21

Kety, S. S., Rosenthal, D., Wender, P. H., et al.: Mental illness in biological and adoptive families of adopted schizophrenics. *Am. J. Psychiatry*, 128: 302–306, 1971.

Rosenthal, D., Wender, P. H., Kety, S. S., et al.: The adopted-away offspring of schizophrenics. *Am. J. Psychiatry*, 128: 307–311, 1971.

Kernberg, O.: Borderline personality organization. *J. Psychoanalytic Assoc.*, 15: 641–685, 1967.

Gunderson, J. G., & Singer, M. T.: Defining borderline patients: An overview. *Am. J. Psychiatry*, 132: 1–9, 1975.